WHO CARES

WHO CARES

EMILY KENWAY

The hidden crisis of
caregiving, and how
we solve it

WILDFIRE

First published in 2023 by
WILDFIRE
an imprint of HEADLINE PUBLISHING GROUP

1

Cataloguing in Publication Data is available from the British Library

Hardback ISBN 978 1 4722 8848 6

Typeset in Minion by CC Book Production

Printed and bound in Great Britain by Clays Ltd, Elcograf S.p.A.

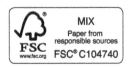

Headline's policy is to use papers that are natural, renewable and recyclable
products and made from wood grown in well-managed forests and other
controlled sources. The logging and manufacturing processes are expected
to conform to the environmental regulations of the country of origin.

HEADLINE PUBLISHING GROUP
An Hachette UK Company
Carmelite House
50 Victoria Embankment
London EC4Y 0DZ

www.headline.co.uk
www.hachette.co.uk

For the overlooked, the unseen, the exhausted;
for those of us who carry this brutal gift;
for the caregivers.

Contents

PROLOGUE
Moonchild   1

CHAPTER 1
On Caregivers: Missing Stories, Missing Solutions   15

CHAPTER 2
On Women: Maidens and Migrants   49

CHAPTER 3
On Technology: Sleepwalking and Seal Pups   93

CHAPTER 4
On Family: Wise Women and the Practice of Kinning   125

CHAPTER 5
On the Mind: Confronting a Convenient Stigma   155

CHAPTER 6
On Freedom: The Lie of the Individual   181

CHAPTER 7
On Work: Breadwinners or Caregivers   215

CHAPTER 8
On Government: Commoning the Horizon   249

CONCLUSION   285

EPILOGUE   301

ACKNOWLEDGEMENTS   305

NOTES   309

Moonchild

At 3am, I'm woken by wailing from upstairs. Well trained by now, I haul my sleep-drugged body out of bed and up to my mum's bedroom. She's lying hunched on her side, shaking, moaning, panting. My days frequently begin this way. Dawn isn't marked by sunrise, but by her pills wearing off. I take her temperature and administer her medication, popping each tablet into her dry mouth and bending a straw to help her swallow them. Then I sit beside her, smoothing my hand back and forth over her arm, telling her it'll pass soon. This may or may not be true. The light around the edges of the curtains turns a paler shade of blue. At around 6am, she's settled and I can go back to bed. At 7am, or thereabouts, her body is racked by retching, hacking coughs. Back in her room, I hold the spittle bowl under her mouth, wiping away the oddly rust-coloured saliva from her lips. Her eyes are almost entirely swollen shut as if she's been in a fight, and her lips protrude forwards in a manner for which many pay hundreds of pounds at cosmetics clinics. This is the effect of the huge dosage of steroids she's on; the rest of what's happening is the effect of the cancer that's killing her.

Who Cares

I wonder what it's like to wake feeling refreshed; I can't remember that sensation anymore. I have a choking pain in my throat that never goes away, a feeling of suffocation in my upper chest. Sometimes when I look in the mirror as I clean my teeth, on the days I have the energy to do that, I notice how my face has begun to cave in and sag, as if the sucking grief of our situation is deflating me from the inside out. Her coughing fit is passing now, so I feed a straw into her mouth again and encourage her to have a few sips of water. I lift her, helping her lean back against her pillows. I try not to notice the uncanny lightness of her body, the way her bones have shifted so much closer to the surface of her skin. Where there was once weight, now there's almost dust. I syringe a few millilitres of liquid morphine into her mouth to ease the coughing and the aching of her joints. I sit for a moment, but then she begins coughing again, and this time it turns into vomiting – not real vomiting, because she can't really eat anymore, but curdling retches that release strange, elastic fluids from somewhere deep inside. I support her as she staggers to the bathroom, wobbly-legged as a colt. The smallest movements have become the greatest effort.

'I hate all this,' she says in a low, angry pant, her hands clutching the sink.

'I know. I'm so sorry it's happening,' I reply, as I often do, rubbing her back. I feel the force of tears behind my eyes and dam them up, refusing to add to her misery by sharing mine. She wants to clean her teeth. It's the one thing, she says, that can still make her feel human. She says it every day, her thoughts starting to loop and repeat as the cancer shrinks and mystifies her world. I know her sense of humour, so I tell her a toothpaste company should use that as an advertising line: *So minty, it makes the dying feel alive!* She laughs and chides me gently, a glimmer of our past relationship when I was the cheeky child and she was the parent. Our roles have largely swapped now.

After she has cleaned her teeth, she tilts her chin upward a little, a modicum of dignity restored. This modicum is needed, because now it's time to change her diaper. The cancer treatment has wrecked her digestive system, leaving her with little control over her bowel movements. The best thing I can do, as I remove the used diaper and sponge away the lurid orange streaks from her body, is talk to her about other things. I bring up the latest political shenanigans and she enjoys expounding on them, the forthrightness of her opinions acting as an antidote to the shame I know she feels at what I'm doing, down here on my knees. I'm the only person she can handle doing this, even though she now has a paid care worker for a couple of hours each day to give me some breathing space. When I was twenty, I had sepsis and very nearly died. All manner of nurses and doctors did all manner of things to me, including a trainee nurse who was my age and did for me what I am now doing for my mum. This is what makes my mum feel more comfortable with me: as I tell her often, I've been an adult in a diaper myself. I understand the shock and shame, the wish to crawl as deep as possible inside your own skin.

Once she's clean, we stagger back to the bed where, in the pause as she enjoys its comfort after so much exertion, I realise that it's already 1pm. We've slipped into a different world where time moves spasmodically, lurching between hours that drag like slow fog and moments that come fast as lightning splitting a tree.

Who Cares

In the grip of a fever, of pain or vomiting, what should be mere minutes stretch until it feels as if our whole life has been this, every breath we've ever taken used up in this relentless war with her breaking body. Care seems to override physics, unhitching our days from the outside world.

My afternoon and evening will look much the same: temperature checking, medication dispensing, diarrhoea wiping, spittle catching, body lifting, sick-bowl washing, eye cleaning, leg creaming, momentarily thinking I should eat something but not really remembering how, temperature checking again, medication dispensing again, diarrhoea wiping spittle catching body lifting sick-bowl washing and on and on and on. Outside on the street, I hear people going about their lives – joggers' fast strides, the rattle of baby buggies, the chatter of couples and neighbours. My phone lights up with news from a friend who's finally moving to Italy with her husband and toddler. They've been hoping to go there for a few years, back to her husband's homeland and a town by the sea, and now it's happening at last. I'm pleased for them, but envious too. I feel I'm living in a long, dark corridor, while my friends outside are chasing the bright successes and joys of a life without death care. In here, our success is when my mum manages to drink half a fortified juice; our joy is the dulled relief when we realise we've managed three hours straight without a vomiting spate. We nod in solidarity with each other as we note the length of the interval. The world is still turning outside, but somehow our axis has got stuck.

When dusk comes, and on days when physical movement is easier, she sits on the edge of the bed, her feet dangling child-like a few inches above the floor. The cancer has shrunk her. I googled why cancer is called 'cancer' once, interested in how this complex and varied disease got its name. As I typed in 'why is cancer called . . .', Google suggested I finish my sentence with the word 'moonchild'. This made no sense to me, so I clicked on it. It turned out to relate to astrology, the believers of which think that a person born under the sign of Cancer is considered a 'moonchild' – that is, their temperament is ruled by the moon. It always comes back to me in the evenings as I look at her sad, swollen face, a haze of white down across her skin, her cheeks pale. She was my mother once; now she has become my moonchild. She tells me in these crepuscular hours how much she doesn't want to die yet, how unhappy she is, and angry too. My mother was a successful career woman before she got sick. When I was young, she often talked about the workplace sexism of the eighties and nineties; how men would call her 'darling' and ask her to make the tea even though she was their equal. She had perfected a withering stare to shut them up. She was on the cusp of retirement when she fell ill. Having worked extremely long hours for decades, she was ready to spend time with friends and family, to travel to places she'd never been, to read and cook and sit in her tiny London back garden in the intermittent sunshine. Instead, she'd been imprisoned in her home or in hospitals. She cries in chirrups, like a small trapped bird, as night sets in. This is the real bitch of care. Not the shit, not the sick, not the syringes and sores and relentless grind of bodily chores. This. Witnessing her suffering, helpless to assuage it. When I look at her, so unhappy and dying, I feel a terrible lurching in my chest. It could be pain, it could be love; I can no longer tell the difference. I stroke her back softly, until she lies down. Her eyes swell shut again as the fluid shifts around her body, sleep a tenuous respite.

She first grew sick in 2016. She had a lump in her neck and was extremely fatigued. The lump was investigated through multiple biopsies and then, one summer's day as I strolled to meet a friend, my hand bouncing over the fence railings along Lincoln's Inn Fields, she telephoned me to say she had the 'all clear'. She did not have cancer. I remember that afternoon as clearly as if I'd trapped it in a globe. It was a bright day and, as she told me the good news, the green grass, the shining black railings, the red of a passer-by's jacket, all seemed to come into sharper focus. But this wouldn't last. Over the following months, as she grew increasingly exhausted, as a chest infection refused to heal, as her iron levels dropped to inexplicably low levels, it became clear that the biopsies weren't omniscient. Then it was confirmed: she had blood cancer after all. A red-haired consultant showed us the scan of her body. They'd injected luminous ink into her veins to show the places where cancer cells were present. There on the screen, her body was lit up all over with yellow splashes like cruel suns. The cancer was in her neck, stomach and groin.

'We're going for the cure,' said the consultant, waving his hands around enthusiastically. 'We're going for the cure,' he repeated.

My mum's case was fairly rare, and we had a sense that the consultants she saw throughout her illness found it interesting and enjoyed the challenge. Movie plots in which people die within weeks of diagnosis or get cured after a few turbulent and vomit-drenched months ran through my mind. But our story would be one largely missing from scripts, and yet far more faithful to so many people's real-life experiences. It would be a long haul of brutal treatment, debilitating side effects and a slow crumbling into eventual death. She was originally diagnosed with leukaemia, but we would soon receive the unwanted revelation that it is possible to have more than one type of blood cancer simultaneously. By the time she was terminally ill, she would have been ravaged by leukaemia and two types of lymphoma, alongside a chronic disease due to a stem-cell transplant she had as treatment for those cancers, and numerous other ailments and problems caused by chemotherapy and other drugs.

My mother was single, my father having left when I was a baby, and my older sister was busy being a mother herself. So, this was how, at the age of thirty-one, I became the default primary caregiver for my mother. Initially, it didn't require too much – she was sick, yes, but we knew this because of the test results, rather than obvious symptoms. But she grew rapidly worse and our definition of a 'good day' downturned sharply throughout the three or so years her illness lasted; at first, it was a day on which she could walk to her local park, about ten minutes from her house; then it became one on which she could do basic chores like hanging up laundry or cooking a simple meal. Eventually, it was one on which she could sit propped up on the sofa for twenty minutes, or perhaps keep down a few spoonfuls of Shreddies. I had some blessed assistance from her out-of-town siblings, my two uncles and aunt, and, in particularly acute months, short shifts from paid help. I learned the practicalities of chronic illness and dying. I learned how to dry someone so they don't get sores, the parts of the body that most need emollient cream, the taut pink shine of a newly bald scalp and the names of more drugs than you can imagine. I learned how post-chemo hair regrowth gives you the fuzzy halo of a pussy willow, and how the best nurses have smiles that seem like a natural quirk of the muscles, rather than a solicitation of a something you can't give. Some of these things were learned during grinding weeks in hospital caused by infections or out-of-control symptoms, others in a relentless trudge at her home in Greenwich, London.

She'd moved there when I was eighteen, to a house one street back from the River Thames. She loved the borough, delighting in its village feel despite its location in London. For a while, her office was west along the Thames, and she found great amusement in taking the river boat to work. On weekends, Greenwich is filled with tourists – foreigners by the coach load, but also Londoners from less idyllic boroughs coming to stroll along the river or visit the bustling craft market. She used to bustle there too, complaining at how slow the tourists were but slowing down herself when she saw something she liked. In summer, she'd escape the crowded centre and go for long walks in the royal park, puffing up the slopes and observing the rose garden change through the seasons. They weren't special days – just ordinary life, lived without much thought. But they became special afterwards, when they were memories of things she could no longer do. Over the years, she grew less and less mobile, parts of her body giving up, others warping, swelling, mottling, drying out. Her Greenwich had become the sliver of paving between her front door and the vehicle parked outside it to take her to hospital appointments. Her house was tall, with an identical row opposite it, and the two together acted as a kind of sound funnel, spinning people's voices from the street up to us in her bedroom. We listened to the world going by, strangers remarking on the architecture or wondering if the river path continued at the other end of the street. They were living their own special moments, and I wondered how many of them knew that. Some of them would realise in time. Like us, they would slip through the looking-glass one day and find themselves bewildered in the land of sickness and care.

They did, but not quite in the way I'd expected: at the start of 2020, two and a half years into my mum's illness, the COVID-19 pandemic took hold. Suddenly, everyone was talking about being walled in, just as we had been for years. I was glad, in a way, that we were being joined in our claustrophobia. It had been a very lonely existence. It also meant there were new ways to connect with people that hadn't existed before, even though so many people had been stuck and isolated long before coronavirus. A charity in the UK set up online video calls for caregivers, and these quickly became a lifeline for me. I'd set my mum up to be as comfortable as possible, a straw in a glass of water poised close to her hand, while I scurried downstairs to share solidarity and pain for an hour with a dozen or so caregivers from all over the country. It seemed ironic, and also a little beautiful, that this most isolating of circumstances could unite people who would otherwise never have met. We were a diverse bag, ranging in age from thirty-something to late seventies, scattered across the country, caring for mothers, partners and children, with vascular dementia, Down syndrome, cancer, Parkinson's, COPD and other conditions. I heard my own desperation echoing back at me in each of their voices. We shared advice, like how to make an adult feel as dignified as possible when their body has reverted to babyhood, and how to navigate complex government bureaucracy in order to access state support. And we shared frustrations, like how our loved one would take out their anger about their vulnerability on us, and how desperately we wanted to know whether 'normal' would always be this strange new life of sickness and care, or if someday things would return to what we'd known before but could barely remember. That single weekly hour of solidarity became so important to me that one week, when I realised at the last minute that, due to an administrative error, the link to join hadn't come through to my emails, I sat in front of my blank computer screen and cried.

Sometimes the people joining the calls changed – being a caregiver is nothing if not unpredictable, and sudden hospitalisations or especially bad days can easily overtake plans – but Deirdre and Anna (not their real names) were devout attendees. Deirdre was caring for her husband in north-west England. She had neatly combed hair framing a long face, made longer by the drag of worry lines around her mouth. She always pronounced her 't's, and chose each word carefully, as if she valued precision. There was an immense sadness to her tone when she spoke. From what I could see behind her in the video, her house was rather big and fancy – polished hardwood floors expanding away into some serious square footage, and elegant furniture that I suspected to be antique. I had the sense that she was terribly alone in a house that was too big for her and her husband, now that their three kids had grown up and moved away.

While Deirdre usually came to the calls with a tense sadness,

Anna came with fury. She'd cared for her heavily disabled son since birth and, now that he was an adolescent, she knew the ins and outs of government bureaucracy like the back of her hand. She vented weekly about all the things the government should be doing but wasn't. Then we'd move on to the specific incidents of that week: someone whose sick husband was hiding his incontinence, another who'd injured her own wrist and couldn't lift her spouse anymore, a third who said little except that they were totally and utterly fed up. When our weekly calls ended, in the short pause between shutting down my laptop and going upstairs to check on my mum, I would think about how absurd it all was. That all of us were miserable and suffocating, and yet the experiences stifling us were an inherent part of human life. As inevitable as the hair growing out of our heads, as the need to breathe or sleep, we can be certain that we'll need to give and receive care in our lives. How could something so natural also be making us choke? And what would a society look like that understood care as an inherent part of human life, instead of a problem in need of a quick fix?

My mother died on 29 September 2020. Over the preceding months, the doctors had looked us in the eyes less and less. Treatment after treatment had failed. I imagined the red-haired consultant moving on to more promising patients, waving his hands around and making enthusiastic pronouncements to the next family in an ever-changing cast of desperate people. Eventually, the doctors said there was nothing else they could do, that she would die, and die soon. There were no more hospital appointments to attend. I took my mum out in a wheelchair whenever the sun was shining, pushing her along the river path and sometimes running to make the chair go faster. She'd yelp with a mixture of jokey annoyance and delight. We discovered that babies were thoroughly entranced by the sight of her, an adult in a pushchair contraption like their own. They'd twist and crane to keep looking back at us, their parents smiling with apologies in their eyes. But within weeks, getting downstairs and out of the house was no longer possible. A palliative care team began to visit regularly, installing a hospital bed in her bedroom, increasing dosages of the drugs designed to numb her body and her mind so that she didn't have to witness her own demise so starkly. She sent me and my sister a final email in broken sentences with her wishes for her funeral, unable to speak about it in person. The palliative care team told me that when people are on the verge of dying, they often seem unconscious, but they can usually hear people talking to them. So on the day she died, I sat beside her for hours, stroking her hand, telling her that my sister and I were going to be fine, thanking her for raising us on her own and encouraging us to become independent-minded people. Eventually, her breaths came further and further apart, then stopped. I watched as the vein in her neck beat weaker. After a few moments, I knew she was no longer with me.

As I sat beside her, waiting for the doctor to come and certify her dead, I was struck by the peculiar fact that, through her stillness as she lay there, in this strange event of her actually having passed away, I was no longer the person I had been for three years or more, this identity I'd been wearing: I was no longer a caregiver.

I'm not woken at 3am by the sound of her wailing anymore. My moonchild mother is not perched there on the side of her bed, wondering sadly why her time came so soon and so cruelly. I'm free to do what I want with my life, but at the price of losing her. But those questions that arose in my mind, about how on earth we've created a world so unable to accommodate and support care, have stayed with me. It's likely I'll care for someone again in my life – a partner, a child, a friend – or that I'll need care myself. The same will be true for you. I miss my blissful ignorance from before my mum got sick – I could never have imagined how hard care would be, how it would reshape everything from the minutiae of my days to my understanding of life. Knowing what I know now, I'm left with two feelings: grief, and the urgent hope that we can remake our world to put care at its heart.

CHAPTER 1

On Caregivers:
Missing Stories, Missing Solutions

'There is a quality even meaner than outright ugliness
or disorder, and this meaner quality is the dishonest
mask of pretended order, achieved by ignoring or
suppressing the real order that is struggling to exist
and to be served.'

– Jane Jacobs[1]

That was my past. If it hasn't been yours yet, the odds are it's
coming. We are only ever temporarily well, temporarily able and
temporarily young. Accident, illness and old age will be part
of our lives at some point, in our own bodies and in those we
love. It follows, then, that we should also expect to be caregivers.

'Care' has many meanings: it's an ethic that suggests loving
attention, and it's a verb that means both 'caring for' – performing tasks and activities that look after someone's needs – and
'caring about' – the emotions of love and affection you feel

when someone is important to you. The two don't always go together, although we often assume they do. The word 'care' is promiscuous: there is care for children, for the sick, impaired and elderly; there is self-care; there is care for the environment and care for non-human animals; there are 'caring' corporations and customer 'care'; and there are care services, from medical assistance in hospitals to volunteers making tea for the lonely elderly.

In these pages, we're concerned with a kind of care for which there is no single word in our vocabulary. We can see this when we consider statistics, articles or political speeches on care in general. They often combine different forms – parenting is lumped together with what I'll be calling *caregiving*, as shorthand for caring for someone who is unable to perform the tasks and activities of daily life without help, such as the elderly, impaired or long-term unwell. Or general parenting is excluded, but they combine paid and unpaid caregiving, as if the experience of a paid care worker is equivalent to that of a wife caring for her ailing husband, a child caring for a mentally unwell father, or me caring for my mother. Every time you hear about paid care workers, supplied by private companies, by the government or by a mixture of the two, pay attention to what's not said; those invisible spaces between shifts, where a family member is constantly on call, always the default, never able to define their own time. Who let the paid care worker into the house for their shift? Who called the local government or company to arrange the care in the first place? Numerous times during the process of researching and writing this book, people asked me what I meant when I said I was writing about caregivers – did I mean care *workers?* Did I mean *social care?* Perhaps I meant the medical professions? Surely I was including general parenting as the paradigmatic caring relationship? No. I meant none of these things. I meant the wraith standing in the corner of the doctor's office or sitting late at night by the sick person's bed; the person hurrying between prescription collections and their own job, wondering when their life took such a turn and how. The individual who is no longer sure they are an individual but has instead become an accessory to someone else's needs. I meant the person who didn't choose to become a caregiver and who must watch as the person for whom they care deteriorates over time despite their loving ministrations. I meant the millions of caregivers who were forgotten when governments were making priority lists for COVID-19 vaccinations, remembering to include 'essential workers' but forgetting the majority of those providing care, the quietly exhausted mass of caregivers. And it is the *majority:* most care in the world today is provided by family and friends, not paid workers, even in wealthier countries with welfare states. Every time someone seemed confused about my topic, I understood the importance of writing about it.

Without words to describe an experience, that experience goes unnoticed. And with caregiving, none of the language fits. It's become common to distinguish between 'informal' caregivers and 'formal' caregivers, the former meaning family or friends who aren't employed to provide that care, the latter being paid care workers who are contracted. But this overlooks the thriving sectors of 'informal-formal' care in many countries, where care has become a job market for undocumented migrants who work without formal contracts. It also suggests a hierarchy of skill that many family caregivers reject. 'Family caregivers', too, is problematic in an age when the concept of family has changed so much and may have little to do with biological or marital ties, something we'll explore more in Chapter 4. We could also question whether we should be naming caregivers at all – isn't it just a natural part of life, to care for those you love when they need it? Why pathologise it by describing it as 'affecting' people and giving it an identity, when it's simply what being a parent/spouse/sibling entails? But without naming the experience, we lose the ability to change it for the better – something sorely needed, as we will see. For example, before second-wave feminism, and before the term 'sexual harassment' was coined, women lacked a way to call out men's lechery in the workplace. It was assumed to be a natural part of life – boys will be boys – and so there was a gap where there should have been a defined concept. In her biography *In Our Time: Memoir of a Revolution,* the prominent second-wave feminist Susan Brownmiller recounted the case of Carmita Wood to illustrate why these kinds of lacunae matter. Wood, a single mother working in Cornell University's nuclear physics department, was forced to leave her job due to the sexual pestering of an eminent professor. When she tried to claim unemployment insurance, she had to give a reason for having left her job. Because there was no socially understood way of describing her experience and why it had led to her resignation, she said she'd left for personal reasons. Consequently, her claim for unemployment insurance was denied. Her experience shows the real-world impacts of gaps in our collective idea-worlds. In this case, second-wave feminists worked hard to change people's perceptions and show that sexual harassment was not just a 'natural' behaviour. By labelling it 'harassment' and attaching that label to ideas of women's right to bodily autonomy and men's accountability, the way we understood the world changed. Women no longer suffered in silence for want of a way to explain their experience.

Today, caregiving remains where sexual harassment once was: missing from our vocabularies and our ideas about how life works and what might need improving. In assembling what we know about this neglected but vital part of our lives, and through combining the rigors of academic research and the pulse of real-life experiences, I hope we can afford caregivers the recognitions, rights and support they need. And remember as we go, 'they' are you in the future. Everything that caregivers experience is coming to you, too. Everything they need, you will need. You'll want to pay attention.

The growing tide of caregiving

For all the media and political discussion of government-provided care services – or the lack thereof – most caregiving in the world continues to be performed by family and friends. The number of people caregiving is astronomical and growing. National data varies significantly between official and unofficial estimates, but at the lowest end, many countries estimate that they are home to millions of caregivers, those overlooked and unpaid family or friends. In the USA, there are approximately 56.4 million caregivers; that's over seventeen per cent of the total population.[2] In the UK, I was one of around 9 million, which is over thirteen per cent of the entire population, and the charity Carers UK believes that 6,000 people become a caregiver each day. Europe-wide, approximately eighty per cent of caregiving is provided by spouses, relatives and friends,[3] while in the Global South, the percentage is higher. This unpaid, under-recognised form of care saves our economies billions each year – around £132 billion in the UK and $470 billion in the USA. In fact, the value of unpaid caregiving exceeds the value of paid care services.[4] If you took all the time that people spend caring solely for those with dementia, you'd get the equivalent of 40 million full-time workers globally, and this is projected to reach 65 million by 2030. Talk of statistics can lose its purchase on our minds. We must remember that facts and predictions mean something tangible for our daily lives. These numbers are the stories of the people we'll encounter through the course of this book: my own story in London, Karen's in Nebraska, Ulla's in Kävlinge, Eric's in Minnesota, Ayesha's in Kathmandu, and more. These numbers mean that, at some point, if you aren't already, you'll be caring for someone you love. Do you know what that will be like? Do you know what you'll need, what you'll lose, how you'll cope?

Those figures may well be underestimates, because many caregivers don't self-identify as such. I didn't recognise that the label 'carer' or 'caregiver' was applicable to me until the second year of my mother's illness. I was just doing what life required. Once I'd accepted this identity, I found myself uncovering a previously hidden world of caregivers' groups, research and campaigning, and a lot of projects trying to provide support. Many people who are technically caregivers don't realise it, because the needs of their loved one have increased gradually over time and so they haven't relabelled the situation in their minds – she's just Mum, he's just Dad, etc. Others deliberately reject the label because of the statement it makes about their relationship to that person. When I meet her online, Katy, a caregiver in her fifties whose husband has motor neurone disease, tells me 'I hated that word to start off with.' In her memoir, *The Cracks that Let the Light In: What I Learned From My Disabled Son*, architect Jessica Moxham opines that 'carer sounds old-fashioned to me, with connotations of older people needing support, of deterioration and medical supplies.'[5] Ulla, who lives in Kävlinge in Sweden and cares for her husband after his stroke, tells me she doesn't see herself as his caregiver because it's less arduous than her experiences of caring for her parents decades ago. Instead, she thinks of herself as his *möjlighetsmakare* – a Swedish word for which there is no English equivalent. She spells it out slowly for me. It means 'possibility maker'.

The problems caused by this ambivalence towards the label of 'caregiver' showed itself on those support calls I joined during the first months of the COVID-19 pandemic. Around ten of us showed up each time, video cameras positioned unflatteringly high or low, Wi-Fi dropping in and out. Often, people shared their confusion about the changes in their relationships with those for whom they were caregivers, the new identities they were forced to try on. Deirdre, whom we met earlier, was caring for her husband, who had dementia: 'He's my husband ... but he's not ... he's not there anymore ... he needs help for everything. It's like having a kid again.'

This self-imposed invisibility stops people being connected with support services. It also perpetuates the long-standing political and social invisibility that makes caregiving so much harder to do on a daily basis. Think about it: many countries around the world now provide rights to *parental* leave – time off employment to birth a child and care for it in its infancy. But a right to *caregivers'* leave – for example, time off to care for a parent with cancer or dementia, or a spouse after a car crash – is a rarity. Equality legislation frequently includes maternity as a protected characteristic, but not caregiving, despite the millions of people affected – a number that will only grow. And when care captures media attention, it's usually to highlight a scandal in a care home or the poor conditions of the underpaid care workforce, not the billions of invisible people providing care 24/7 in their homes. Although I'm mainly concerned with caregivers who have longer-term responsibilities than might arise from, say, a loved one needing a week to recover from a run-of-the-mill operation or virus, our lives are still punctuated by moments in which we need to either receive or give care. Our bodies are terrifyingly breakable, much as we may wish to pretend otherwise. Having structures in place in our lives that mean, when the time comes, we'll be able to provide or receive care, is surely only common sense. But that's far from our current reality.

Karen is in her fifties and lives in Nebraska, USA, with her husband, who's recently retired. She bursts on to my laptop screen five minutes late, having slept later than usual, pulling a blue bandana over her hair. She's one of those people to whom you warm immediately, her face expressive in its changeable emotions, her exclamations searching for shared experiences. For the next hour and a half, she lays before me the details of her circumstances. Karen is a typical example of a caregiver today – and of what becoming a caregiver does to a life. She is caring for her parents, aged eighty-four and eighty-five, both of whom have dementia, though her mother's is substantially worse than her father's. Karen is their only daughter, and what Karen perceives as her brother's absence of hands-on support, despite his being retired while Karen still works, is typical of caregiving patterns: there's a hierarchy of care in which adult daughters are more likely to provide care than adult sons, regardless of who has more time on their hands.

The hours she spends taking care of her parents have varied, but during the height of the COVID-19 pandemic in 2020, she estimates it was around twenty-five hours a week. She cooks and cleans for them. She tries to keep their hoarding tendencies at bay to limit their confusion as they navigate their home. For a while, she was putting her mother's medication into day-of-the-week boxes, but then discovered her mum was moving them around within the box, so now she has the pharmacist make them into blister packs instead. She doesn't yet need to bathe them, but 'it's coming', she says. And Karen should know: in her professional life, she's an occupational therapist who specialises in working with the elderly. Her life is permeated by breaking minds and bodies, both at home and at work. This, she says, makes her caregiving role both easier and harder: she knows what to do when others might not (like when she knew the pharmacist could make bespoke blister packs of medication), but she also recognises what she's failing to do far more acutely that you or I might. Her ready exclamations of solidarity when I share some of my experiences are punctuated by sudden tears as she explains how hard her life feels.

The care world is one about which few people know until they're forced to step into it. If you look, you'll find thousands of message boards, virtual and in-person groups, forums, support lines and advice services. And in all of them, you'll find the same themes repeated: caregivers sending out distress flares as they suffer financially, emotionally, socially and physically due to their situation. Karen is experiencing all these types of suffering. 'I think I've lost half the income I could have made because of how many shifts I'm saying no to,' she tells me. Study after study has found that caregiving causes severe financial strain. In the USA, caregivers lose thirty-three per cent of their income on average, and approximately eleven per cent quit work altogether because of their caregiving responsibilities, like I did towards the end of my mum's life.[6] Overall, lost income due to family caregiving in the USA is estimated to be around $522 billion *each year*.[7] A fifth of caregivers report financial strain as a result of caring responsibilities,[8] which can be because of loss of work, but also because of the extra costs of care, including travel costs, medications, devices and so on. Definitions of care often involve words like 'love' or 'affection' while conveniently omitting its material costs. Karen's loss of income won't just affect her finances now, but in the future, too, when she herself needs care: women who reduce hours or stop working altogether have substantial pension losses.

Katy, who said she hated being called a caregiver at first, is 4,000 miles away from Karen but facing similar issues. She cares for her husband, Mark, who has a form of motor neurone disease, and also for her mum, who's had several small strokes. Now in their fifties, Katy and Mark have been together since they were teenagers and she still speaks of him with an endearing giddiness. Before she had to give up working to care for Mark, Katy was a teacher. She tells me: 'I did all the right things – I had savings, I always put a bit of my salary away. But now I can't work, and when I think about my old age, basically, I'm screwed.'

Karen and Katy's social lives have both taken a hit too. Katy says she has a 'typical carer story', because she's lost friends through not being able to go to things like she could in the past. Karen, meanwhile, is dejected and tired: 'Oh, my social life is terrible, I don't do anything,' she sighs. She feels her friends think she should put her parents in a home, but says: 'I do inherently think it's kind of disrespectful. If they don't want to go to a home, just because our culture says that's where everyone goes, they don't have to.' Meanwhile, along with her bank balance and her social life, her mental and physical health are suffering. She tells me she's gained a lot of weight and that her daughter frets about her wellbeing, the fear of loss and sickness ricocheting down the generations. 'I just feel so overwhelmed and tired with everything,' she says about the idea of going for a walk. Studies abound showing that caregivers experience higher rates of heart disease, high blood pressure, diabetes and depression.[9] When I ask if caregiving has affected her psychologically, her face contorts immediately and her answer comes out in such a choked whisper that I have to replay my recording of our conversation several times to be certain of her words: 'Like crazy.' I'm reminded of the lines in a poem by Adrienne Rich in which she explores the death of the self that can occur when life is wholly subsumed by caring for others: 'For you are not a suicide, but no one calls this murder.'[10] Karen's been thinking about going to counselling. It doesn't help that her marriage is also affected by the situation; she has no energy to give to the relationship, she says, and she can tell her husband 'wants me to take care of myself a bit'.

The extremity of caregiving is made worse when there's no time off from its responsibilities. The last time Katy had some time off caring for someone, it was a few hours to go to a hospital appointment about the eye in which she'd previously suffered a detached retina. She describes having a cup of coffee while she waited. Not quite a holiday, then. Katy should be an outlier, but she isn't. According to charity Carers UK, one in four caregivers they surveyed hadn't had a day off in a year, and a quarter hadn't had one in five years.[11] If caregiving were a job, this would be a scandal. In many countries in the world, we don't even know how stressed, depressed and anxious caregivers are, simply because no one is asking them.

How did Karen and Katy, and all the millions of other caregivers, end up in this state? Broadly speaking, there are six reasons why life is so hard for these invisible millions today. Our brief tour of them begins in the 1939–45 war. It's often discussed as the crucible in which the welfare state as we know it was born, but it had another important effect on care less often noted in mainstream commentary. In the USA, around 2,000 conscientious objectors were assigned to work in understaffed mental institutions during the war.[12] For the first time, people from outside that world were seeing what went on behind its closed doors and barred windows. In May 1946, some of those men got an exposé in *Life* magazine describing the abject conditions in government-run facilities, leading to a flurry of reports and then the establishment of the National Mental Health Foundation in Philadelphia.[13] Comparable developments occurred in the UK: in 1967, Barbara Robb published *Sans Everything: A Case to Answer*, a book detailing the poor and abusive care to which she'd seen elderly women subjected in long-stay hospitals. Hot on its heels, a series of scandals about the abuse of the mentally unwell, disabled or elderly in institutions engulfed the British press. At Ely Hospital in Cardiff, Wales, patients had been assaulted, refused medical treatment, subjected to lengthy seclusions, and had their food stolen by staff;[14] similar allegations abounded from other institutions. The era of institutionalisation was ending. What began in the aftermath of the war turned into mass deinstitutionalisation throughout the mid-to late twentieth century, with hundreds of thousands of people moved back into the community. 'A new era of residential and group homes, day care facilities and independent living within mainstream communities began,' writes historian Simon Jarrett.[15]

But there was a problem. Deinstitutionalisation didn't only occur because of the scandals and campaigns. Governments liked it because it promised to save money. It was assumed that 'care in the community' would be less costly to the public purse than running (quality) institutions. This underlying aim of saving money meant that funding for community-based support was insufficient. Nearly fifty years after the Ely Hospital scandal, the director of a disability charity in the UK said: 'People with a learning disability may no longer be segregated by buildings, but social isolation is still widespread – and access to friendships and relationships, outside of formal care or support services, may be even worse now than it was then.'[16]

Our second stop on this brief tour is a natural follow-on from our first: care in the community, rather than in institutions, has meant more reliance on family. But shifts in family composition have also occurred, and they don't marry with this reliance. The overall trend is for families to be smaller today than they were in the past. The average woman marrying in her teens or early twenties in the 1890s experienced ten pregnancies – far more than today.[17] With fewer children being born, we end up with a skewed 'old-age dependency ratio' – that is, the proportion of people aged sixty-five and older in relation to the population of 'working age'. My own family bears out this trend: my mother's mother was one of six, she herself was one of four, and I'm one of two. China's former one-child policy has wreaked havoc on its old-age dependency ratio. In its largest city, Shanghai, nearly a third of the residents are older than sixty.[18] In 2021, China announced that couples would be permitted to have up to three children (having already increased the allowance to two children) in order 'to actively respond to the ageing of the population'.[19] One citizen writing on Weibo saw it as too little too late, and was quoted by the *Guardian* as saying: 'I myself am a product of the one-child policy. I already have to take care of my parents. Where would I find the energy to raise more than two kids?'

More than a quarter of Japan's population are over sixty-five,[20] while the USA will have more older adults than children by 2035, a situation described by one demographer as 'the graying of America'.[21] This will affect the elderly and their few geographically proximate adult children, but it will also affect much younger kids, who will need to become family caregivers. Estimates for the UK from the University of Nottingham have suggested that around 800,000 children aged eleven to eighteen are 'young caregivers'.[22] In the USA, the last major survey found more than a million young caregivers aged eight to eighteen, but this is thought to be an underestimate, partly because parents had to give their consent for children to respond to the survey, and partly because that survey took place in 2004, before the opioid epidemic took hold.[23] For many countries, there has never been a survey of how many children's lives are affected by caregiving. Basically, there are loads of older people, and too few younger people. It's likely that you have far fewer siblings than your ancestors did; this means you're going to need to do a lot more caregiving (or be judged as heartless).

These smaller families are also likely to live further apart than they did historically. This is due to several factors, including the introduction of pensions, which create economic independence in the elderly, enabling them to live alone, and also increased migration for work opportunities, something that particularly affects those in the Global South and in rural areas. Lots of caregiving is provided by spouses, so increased divorce rates mean many older people are without that 'built-in' caregiver, putting more pressure on siblings or children. These are problems that pay no heed to borders. In Russia, the co-residence of family members that characterised the Soviet era has ended, and now that migration is possible, more people are moving abroad for work.[24]

Our third stop now quickly comes into view: even when

there are plenty of children *and* they live in proximity, the era of assuming the daughters in a family will be unemployed and available to provide free care is long gone. Increasing numbers of women now participate in the labour market, with numbers in the USA doubling between 1975 and 2016, and in the UK rising by over a third from 1975 to 2017.[25] Few issues can be so similar and unifying across such wide geographical, cultural and political terrain, but when it comes to the family's role in caregiving, we're dealing with a very human problem, from London to Nebraska, Nepal to Moscow.

The human infrastructure of caregiving is dwindling, yet it's needed now more than ever before: advances in medicine mean that we live longer, but this also means we live longer when we're sick. This is the fourth reason for the modern state of care. Today, babies born with impairments have longer life expectancies than they did historically. Dementia cases are growing exponentially: according to the World Health Organization, there are currently 50 million people suffering from dementia worldwide, with 10 million new cases each year. Or take Parkinson's disease: in the USA, the number of people living with it has nearly doubled since 1978,[26] and its prevalence is expected to double in the UK by 2065.[27] Diseases like these can be managed in the long term, extending people's lives – but that comes with a care requirement attached. And when we hear tales of people 'beating' cancer, it's pronounced like a single plot line, when in fact it has a deeply distressing subplot: the long tail of chronic symptoms that come after harsh treatments. Academics project that in 2050, the 'oldest-old' population (those aged over eighty-five) will be triple what it is today. We are standing on the shore, watching a tsunami of chronic and acute conditions gathering out at sea, seemingly blind to what that'll mean for our lives: we will all be providing care.[28]

Combine all this with our fifth cause: the insidious trend to shift medical support from hospitals to homes. Inpatient stays – both in terms of being admitted at all and the length of stay if you are admitted – are decreasing.[29] Advances in medical devices over recent decades mean that complex tasks and processes are much more likely to be done in the home, by you. The US think tank Third Way called for a national strategy for caregivers in 2017, citing cases like that of Angela Goodhope of Mapleton, Iowa. Every day, Angela must clean and disinfect her teenage daughter's central line (a catheter delivering medicine into a large vein to treat blood cancer). This disinfection is vital in the true sense of the word: if the central line becomes infected, deadly bacteria can enter a vein next to her daughter's heart.[30] It's symptomatic of the medicalisation of the home, and therefore the work required of family caregivers. Eric is in his forties and lives in Minnesota, where he cared for his husband, Scott, who died of cancer in August 2019. 'You have to become all of these armchair versions of medical professions when you're caring for someone and you don't have the expertise,' he tells me. 'You're just trying to do the best that you can by talking to the care team, but then you have to do it all.'

Even when your loved one is in hospital, you may need to be there. Jessica Moxham writes that there aren't enough nurses to keep an eye on her son, so she and her husband are expected to be there all the time: 'We live close to the hospital and so they allow us to go and sleep . . . in our own beds, on the under-standing that we will return early the next morning.' Likewise, during my mum's long stints of hospitalisation, I would wash her, deal with her drip machines and adjust her oxygen supply. I'd be there before going to my job and I'd return after, becoming familiar with asking security guards to let me out of the hospital building in the small hours of the night.

Finally, since the financial crash of 2008, many governments have implemented devastating cuts to publicly funded services, including care. This puts more pressure on caregivers in the home, whether by reducing their access to paid care workers with whom to share the load, or closing down day and respite centres that provide vital time off care, whether to recuperate or to earn. Taking all this in, a looming catastrophe of care is hard to deny.

The uncomfortable truth about care

This catastrophe is often discussed as a purely political one. But it's also personal, and some of those personal aspects aren't easily solved by government funding or different insurance arrangements. The extent to which caregivers are harmed by their experiences varies according to their relationship with the person for whom they're caring. Through the course of caring for my mum, our dynamic shifted. We'd never been your classic parent–child combination – my mum struggled with depression when I was a child and continued to have difficulties navigating some aspects of life. But through her sickness, as her body disintegrated and aged, her personality shifted strikingly. She became childlike. Her emotional regulation, which had never been very good, worsened; tantrums, sudden outbursts and panics appeared or were amplified. She began referring to herself as 'little', to parts of her body as 'little' too, and she even seemed to take on a younger posture – legs swinging from the sides of furniture, feet turned slightly inwards when I helped her to shower, a doddering but needful uncertainty like that of a child. The term 'ambiguous loss' was coined by therapist Dr Pauline Boss in 1999. It's used for types of loss that include a combination of absence and presence. Specifically, Boss uses it for dementia – when a person is physically present but psychologically absent – and for missing people – when a person is physically absent but emotionally present. When a parent becomes very sick, and stops being 'the person they were', both in themselves and in relation to you, their child, there is a loss, an absence, despite their presence. This loss is felt in every interaction, a jarring cognitive dissonance, the absence of safe harbour at the precise moment that life is bringing you the raging waters of disease and death.

While I felt a confused and ambiguous sense of loss, Karen's situation is uncomfortably clear-cut. I wrote earlier that caregiving comprises both 'caring about' and 'caring for', but this isn't quite accurate. Sometimes, there's a lot in column B and very little in column A. Karen describes her father as a mean man with 'a mood problem'. She says he's always been cruel to her, putting her down, being disrespectful. Before her parents got sick, she didn't allow him to come around to her house because of these issues. And now she must care for him. A few days before we spoke, she'd decided: she would leave her parents' house whenever he was nasty to her. She knits her fingers together as she explains, and I get the sense that it takes a great deal of strength from her to uphold this boundary. Professor Emily K. Abel interviewed daughters caring for their disabled parents in 1980s Los Angeles. In the resultant book, she writes that caregiving 'revived powerful elements of the original parent–child relationship' and that 'issues they assumed had been fully resolved suddenly re-emerged. Several women were shocked by the intensity of the feelings this experience provoked. Although a few viewed caregiving as an opportunity to master old conflicts, many stated that they simply slipped back into old patterns.'[31] These emotional complexities of caregiving are as much part of our looming catastrophe as macrotrends on population growth or austerity economics.

But contrast Karen's emotional strife with Eric's story. His facial expression when he speaks about his husband Scott is beatific. Before we spoke, I'd been re-reading the emails he sent me, and when he arrived at our interview, I called him Scott by accident. I apologised profusely and he assured me that it was fine; he's still 'Scott's Eric', he said, and it made him feel close to him. In February 2015, they were on their honeymoon in Miami, hoping to have a long and happy life together. In March, Scott was diagnosed with cancer. Throughout his sickness, Scott would check how Eric was doing, despite his own discomforts. He'd persuade Eric to go for runs because he knew it helped his wellbeing. Although Eric was Scott's caregiver, Scott cared for him, too, and this mutual yet necessarily differing exchange seems to have made Eric's experience very different from those

trying to provide care in more emotionally fraught circumstances. Think of your relationships with family members: all
the ways in which you do and don't get along, the shared senses
of humour or the repetitious jibes, the innate similarities and
fundamental differences. All of these travel with you into the
realm of caregiving. There, you must do everything kindly and
patiently, regardless of the nature of your relationship. Love is
a messy thing; so too, then, is care.

Leave no caregiver behind

Things are bad for Karen, but stepping back, she's coming up
roses compared to caregivers in other parts of the world. Karen
has a home, she has some savings, and she has a profession that
earns her good money (when she's able to work). For those at
the bottom of the world economy, that would be a dream scenario. Anil Patil is the founder and executive director of Carers
Worldwide, an extraordinary organisation with an extraordinary origin, the kind that gives you faith that a better world is
possible. Growing up in a conservative and 'totally religious'
family in India, Anil was expected to embark on a sensible
career. And he did, training as a veterinarian and getting a
permanent contract that would set him up for a good life with
a reliable pension. But he hated it. Being a veterinarian for farm
animals was a sad business and, after eighteen months, Anil quit,
seeking something that would bring 'happiness and satisfaction,
something meaningful'. He had no money and his parents were
deeply unimpressed by this seemingly impetuous change of

heart, but after much searching and barely getting by, he found an internship in a development charity and began learning about their work among the impoverished rural villages of India. One day, he saw a woman in the throes of a mental health crisis. She was naked, dirty and lashing out. Anil wanted to help her, but it wasn't within the remit of the organisation's work. He thought of her often, though, unable to sleep knowing she was without help. Eventually, he left that organisation and began working on mental illness in rural areas, for which there was almost no provision. Through this work, he often encountered the family caregivers of mentally unwell people, and they would ask him the same questions over and over again: 'Why has this happened to us? What happens to them if I die tomorrow?' He realised the family members themselves were under huge pressure but, for now, his interest remained with the patients.

Some years later, he met and married Ruth, and they flew back to her native UK to have their first child. Their daughter was born with tethered spinal cord syndrome, requiring extensive medical intervention. They decided to remain in the UK, where there was sufficient support, and there they had their second child, another daughter, who was born with Down syndrome. Caregiving had collided with his life; now that seed of concern for caregivers, sown years before in rural India, would begin to grow. In person, Anil carries himself with a benevolent humility. He speaks softly but with total precision – accurate statistics fly off his tongue with ease, and when he describes extreme hardship, he says it with a compassionate matter-of-factness that begs no sympathy, yet stands in knowing solidarity with the raw sufferings that life can entail.

'As you can imagine,' he says in this characteristic manner, 'when [our second daughter] was born, it was quite challenging. The same questions went through my mind – why us? What did we do? She is very bright; she's beautiful and funny. It's a privilege to have her. She's enriching our lives. But without the support of friends and family, and of the professional services available here, I don't think we'd have coped well.'

This was the moment that the two parts of Anil's life – his work and his family – came together: a fortunate alignment for the hundreds of thousands of caregivers whom his work has now helped. Anil used his own savings to go on a research trip throughout India and South Africa to understand the issues faced by caregivers in low- and middle-income countries. It was the first time in their lives that anyone had asked these overlooked people about themselves. 'Carers would say, "This is the first time anybody has seen me here, recognised me, even my family members. Nobody has asked me questions like these – have I got food? How am I sleeping? How is my health?" They were crying and crying, they couldn't contain it. They were holding so much in them.'

Anil's research formed the foundation of the new organisation he set up, Carers Worldwide, which has now brought that same recognition and vital support, to caregivers in Nepal, India and Bangladesh. The problems he sees are the same as those Karen is experiencing, only amplified. Financial losses become destitution; social ostracisation and romantic neglect become total abandonment by husbands; physical impacts go untreated and mental health slips into crises. 'The issues of carers are the same everywhere, but the scale of the issues is different,' he tells me. Elineca Ndowo, based in Tanzania, works for ADD International, a charity that tackles discrimination against disabled people in the Global South. 'It is very challenging,' she tells me about life for caregivers there. 'They will live a very low economic condition, a very poor life.' Carers Worldwide's strapline is 'leave no carer behind', an aspiration that we are tragically far from realising.

Love, reciprocity, obligation

If caregiving is so awful, why do we do it? If it doesn't necessarily involve love, what, then, is it? What is the nature of this thing that pervades our lives, that will shape chapters of yours, that is on the brink of global catastrophe? Of course, caregiving isn't uniformly awful. The degree of awfulness is contingent on many factors, some of which have already been explored. As we'll see in due course, much can also be gleaned and learned from being a caregiver. Just as some relationships grow more fractious in the crucible of care, so others cleave together. In the interviews for this book, and in personal interactions with friends who sought advice during their own unexpected-yet-predictable caregiving situations, I was struck by the difference between caregiving situations involving an adult child caring for their parent, and those involving someone caring for their spouse. Often, the former were far more difficult, involving complex dynamics and heart-breaking histories, whereas the latter seemed to maintain – and even, at times, enhance – the love between the pair. When I asked adult-children caregivers what words they'd use to describe caring, they invariably made suggestions steeped in negativity: *exhausting, miserable, depressing, a nightmare.* Eric, who held his love for Scott so warmly across his countenance, chose *illuminating.* Caregiving can be all and any of those things. What it can't be, however, is avoided.

Broadly speaking, we care today for three reasons: love, reciprocity and cultural norms. The first reason is obvious; we love someone, so we care for them (assuming our situation allows us to – a degree of material security and civil freedom is necessary). Despite appearances, Karen is certainly caring for her dad out of love, albeit a profoundly painful inflection of it: 'I still want him to like me,' she weeps when I ask her why she does it. Often related to love, many people explain their caregiving as being due to the care once provided to them by the sick or elderly loved one, or because they may inherit property or money from that person once they die. In these instances, it's a kind of exchange.

Relatedly, just as there is a norm that parents care for infant children, so there is a norm of adult children caring for elderly parents, or wives doing so for husbands. Professor Evelyn Nakano Glenn of the University of California uses the term 'status obligation' to capture this idea, meaning the duties assigned to all those in a particular status, for example, wife, mother, daughter, daughter-in-law (you may notice these are all woman-related words, something to which we will return in Chapter 2). This, she explains, is different to the norm of reciprocity, in which you incur obligations as debts for gifts or services you've received. Nor are status obligations the same as contractual obligations, which are (in theory) incurred by voluntarily entering into an agreement to provide services. This is one of the reasons Glenn views much caregiving as coercive – purely because you are the daughter, the daughter-in-law or the wife, you must give substantial portions of your life energy to caregiving, regardless of your own desires.[32] In some countries and states, the obligation of children to care for their elderly parents has been enshrined in law. These 'filial responsibility' laws exist in several US states and many Canadian provinces, and in other countries including Germany, France and Taiwan. They usually focus on financial support rather than physical, especially when a parent is impoverished, though they are rarely enforced.

Cultural obligation doesn't mean that people are content to be caregivers. Racial stereotypes that some groups, such as Asian women, are more amenable to caregiving roles are brought into question when researchers ask them how they feel. In a study exploring the experiences of Taiwanese women caring for their in-laws, the discontent is clear. One woman, caring for her mother-in-law, explained: 'I am too tired. I think I should hire an aid, or I would collapse before she does. My mood is very low. I don't know how long the suffering will last.' Another said that the anxiety caused by being a caregiver meant she had to visit the doctor: 'I suffered from dizziness, fainting, soreness and aches throughout my whole body.' The research found that married women expected to care for their in-laws and saw it as a time-honoured role for them to fulfil. But it was still incredibly difficult and created a sense of entrapment: 'Now, I just live a "numb" life . . . every day is like a circle.'[33]

There is no solution without caregivers

If this were an in-person discussion about care, rather than a book, someone would surely by now have raised the idea that this can all be solved by having sufficient government-funded care services, often called 'social care' because it's care that's 'socialised', meaning organised at a collective level, usually by government. As I describe the facts of obligation, in law or in practice, around the world, a well-meaning interlocuter would volley back at me: *But what about Sweden? Norway? These countries where they have taken the burden off the family and made caregiving a responsibility of government!*

For the millions of caregivers around the world, and especially those in countries with substantial government-provided care, this is a frustrating assumption that bears little relation to reality. If this is a solution to the problems I've described, why does Line, who cares for an adult son with impairments in Norway, a country that has extensive support, tell me that what she needs is less struggle to access that support, that she misses her freedom and that her life is like 'living with no dreams'? And why does nearly a fifth of Sweden's adult population provide familial care, with almost a third of those people caring for more than ten hours a week?[34]

Katy and her husband don't have state help in the form of paid care workers coming in to support them. Instead, they have Katy's 'free' labour and are living off her husband's pension and a paltry government benefit for caregivers (at the time of writing, £67.60 week). But if they did have government-provided care services, Katy would still need to be doing many of the things she's doing. This is something people don't realise. Even in those countries where there's considerable government provision, kin caregivers are still necessary. They support the person who needs care by helping them to navigate the system, to advocate for their rights, to understand and select from the options available, and to oversee the care provided. Their role is crucial and inextricable from good care. Not to mention the fact that many people who require care are non-verbal or have cognitive issues; having a trusted advocate is vital. 'What happens if I have dementia and can't advocate for myself, even if I wanted to?' points out Kirsty Woodard from Ageing Without Children (AWOC), a project she created to highlight the risks facing the growing segment of the world's population who don't have the offspring on which our care systems rely. 'That's what people's adult children are doing . . . they're making sure someone goes around to give their mum a bath. And if no one does . . . they're on the phone to someone, going, "Why hasn't someone been around to give my mum a bath? Why did they only stay thirty seconds? What's going on?" That's what adult children are doing.'

While some of these functions could be performed by well-trained workers, others require long-standing relationships to be effective. Towards the very end of my mother's life, her speech became warped. It was as if her mouth couldn't form the vowels and consonants it needed, making only loose twisting sounds. A palliative nurse was with me for a few minutes one morning and we were discussing some medication when my mother interjected. The nurse looked at me askance – she had no idea what my mother had said. All she heard was, no doubt, a strange, twisting collection of pitches, an impressionist's sentence. But I understood exactly what my mum said. She was telling us where to find a spare box of her steroid pills, downstairs in the kitchen. I understood because I'd known her for thirty-something years. Because I knew the specific ways she constructed sentences, the rhythms and emphases, and the type of person she was (always on the ball, and keen on giving orders!). The intimate involvement of someone who has a relationship of trust and knowledge is irreplaceable.

To focus on government services as the solution to care is to fail to understand how care actually happens as a daily practice. This is not to say that government services are irrelevant; of course, sufficient provision of free, quality care support alleviates the strain on caregivers. But in political debates about the precise forms, funding pots and structures of those services, kin caregivers are too often omitted or assumed to be a vestige of arrangements that can be superseded. Tell me, when a loved one suddenly needs care, how long will it take to get a paid worker to come regularly to the house? Someone must be there in the meantime. Will there be gaps in between shifts? Someone must be there in those gaps. How will the care worker get into the house? Someone must be able to open the door. If, like with my mother, a lock-box is installed on the outside of the house for nurses and suchlike to let themselves in, someone still has to approve its installation, someone has to get extra keys cut, someone has to be there when it is installed. And who will check that the person in need of care has been bathed? That the medication delivery has come on time? If a paid care worker is tasked with these things, what if they don't do it? Many care workers are brilliant; some will, inevitably, be less so. Who will check? Will there always be two care workers at your home at the precise moment that a four-handed job, like lifting to change an adult diaper, is needed? What if the person who needs care – your partner, your parent, your child – doesn't want outsiders doing it? Will you ignore them, override their autonomy and dignity? If your care plan entails two shifts from care workers a day and it works just fine until your elderly father gets an infection and needs continuous care, who's going to provide that care when it's needed out of nowhere? Are you envisaging a reserve army of paid care workers who simply wait for emergencies? In the vague notion that outside services – provided by the private sector, government or various other forms like co-operatives – can offer care if only they're funded enough, there seems to be an assumption that you'll get to be there for the *nice* things, but not the *necessary* things. Sickness, impairment and disease don't work like that; very sick bodies are not manageable or obedient to routines. Understanding the bodily reality of care immediately requires a different approach.

Perhaps most strikingly overlooked is the issue of love. In the final stages of my mother's life, nurses and assistants came to the house. They would come twice a day, once mid-morning and once mid-afternoon, to help give her bed baths and change her incontinence wear, check her medication and make any necessary changes. They were brisk, skilled and highly efficient women who had seen it all before. One of them wore a watch pinned to her breast pocket engraved with *Carpe diem*. I can't remember how long their visits were, but they were certainly no longer than an hour. Even if they'd been far longer, I'd still have wanted to be there most of the time, simply because it was the end of my mother's life and I loved her. Would you miss out on the penultimate squeeze of a loved one's hand? Their last smile? The final opportunity to share aloud the memory of that day in early summer when we walked to the park for the last time, when she wore the blue dress she'd just bought even though she said it was silly to buy new things so close to, well, *you know*, and you insisted on having ice cream together because you were desperate to see her smile, and you handed her a huge cone, two scoops, already starting to drip, *Delicious* she said, and all across her face you could see that yes, she was feeling alive for once, and so were you, together in a brief bubble of forgetting, a final outing of joy before the inevitable?

The majority of care in the world is still provided by family members, and that's not solely for lack of government replacements. It's because of all the reasons described: because of love, because of reciprocity, because of cultural norms and because it's simply necessary due to the *unpredictable and bodily reality of care*. When we focus on external services as the solution without including the much-needed changes for caregivers, we erase the crucial contribution of those 'someones'. In doing so, we perpetuate the selective blindness that makes their oft-miserable task even more miserable.

Time to bear witness

This selective blindness was stripped away when COVID-19 began wreaking its havoc in the world. As I explained earlier, by then my mum had already been sick for some time. Life was small, sad and airless. Our concerns and conversations revolved around hospital appointments, medications, and the dangers of the outside world for someone with an immune system rendered non-existent by treatment after brutal treatment. Considering this abject situation, it was a relief to find everyone else suddenly isolated too, living with constant anxiety about illness. Tracy lives in a wooded area of Michigan with her boyfriend. She cared for her mother, who died of a heart problem a few years ago, and now she's caring for her father, who has dementia. When we speak, she tells me that what she finds stressful is the lack of control over her days and her future: 'I don't know where it's going to go, I don't know what's going to be happening a year from now, I don't know how I'm going to be handling it mentally . . . just the unknown.' She could be talking about COVID; she's talking about care.

With everyone suddenly alighting in our bewildering parallel world, many caregivers thought that, at last, some positive change might come to pass. Yet still, caregiving remained a peripheral concern. As op-eds and political chat shows discussed the difficulties of self-isolating and the newfound sense of entrapment shared by all, the billions of caregivers around the world saw their already-troubled lives become even harder. Day centres and related services closed, and paid care workers were unable to go to people's homes, removing caregivers' support systems. The groups and centres initiated by Carers Worldwide in Nepal and India closed. Karen became so terrified of her parents falling, needing to go to hospital and catching COVID-19 there, that she was anxious every time they climbed the stairs. I stressed about how to get groceries to my mum safely, not knowing in the early stages of the pandemic whether the virus could be transferred by touch. A survey looking at the global impact of the pandemic on caregivers found that people were spending more hours caring than before.[35] Nearly two thirds said the pandemic had made caregiving harder, and many found that its most challenging impact was the inability to take a break from caregiving.[36] Newspapers were filled with the trials of home-schooling; far less attention was dedicated to those who had already been trapped in their lives, and now were even more so. Caregiver poverty worsened, from the UK, where caregivers were disproportionately likely to use food banks[37], to India, where local NGO Samuha had to run an emergency appeal to distribute grain kits. It was forgotten in the endless chatter about 'getting back to normal' that some people's 'normal' had been unbearable to begin with. Everyone was desperate to move on, as if there was a hallowed future ahead in which disease doesn't exist – and neither, then, would the need to care.

It's easy to turn away from the inconspicuous tragedy of care, until it comes to your own doorstep. Projections for the future are bleak if things continue as they are. We face a looming dystopia. But we can avoid it – if we make the right changes in the right ways. To do that, we must first bear witness to the reality of caregiving today.

CHAPTER 2

On Women: Maidens and Migrants

I am not beautiful,
Yet, I am the most wanted woman.
I am not rich,
Yet, I am worth my weight in gold.
I might be dull, stupid,
Dirty and mean,
Yet, all doors are open for me.
I am a welcome guest.
All of the elite compete for me.
I am a maid.

> – Arvo Lindewall, 1925[1]

If I had to choose only one word to describe my mother, it would be 'feminist'. She was a woman who took no prisoners and had no need of a man to shape her life. She taught my sister and me, both implicitly and explicitly, that our lives were *ours,* not to be defined by gendered roles. There was no question of some careers being off limits because of our femininity; life was there to be shaped by our choosing. It was a shock, then, to find myself in my early thirties and suddenly required to step off a careerist path and into the classic storyline of women's history: care. You see, it's not a coincidence that I'm a woman and I'm writing a book about caregiving. Today, for all our advances, women are still the primary caregivers of sick, elderly and impaired people around the world today. In my family, it was less obvious than in others, because I have no father present and my sibling is a sister, so there were no men to shirk care within our direct family unit. Thankfully, I also had helpful uncles. But if this book succeeds at giving you a new lens through which to view the world, one that foregrounds caregiving in your perspective, you'll start to experience a drip-feed of disappointment as you realise that the caregivers around you are almost all women. Try asking people at a party or after-work drinks which of them has a sick or impaired family member, and who it is that cares for them. The answers will be wives, mothers, sisters and aunts. You won't be popular, but you'll be disabused of the idea that we've achieved gender equality. Often, the answers you'll receive will come with a rationale about why it's the women rather than the men providing care – it's because of his location, the nature of his work, that he's not very good at 'that sort of thing', and so on. I'm sure all those things are often true, and I'm also sure that for every specific reason given for a man not performing familial care, there's a woman who never even got to put her reasons forward. There is a kind of collective gullibility taking place whereby we've decided to believe in these 'reasons' as facts, instead of choices. It's exactly the kind of world that the feminists of my mother's generation thought they were ending.

But as much as I may want to rail against the gender inequality of care, I'm also acutely conscious that the story of care is not one in which all women have the same experience. There are two types of women when it comes to care. The category into which a woman falls has determined whether she needs to fight to be freed from family caregiving obligations, or alternatively to fight to care for her kin at all. This was made very real to me during one of my mother's many stints in hospital. I can't remember when it was – as any long-term caregiver will tell you, after a while, the roller coaster of emergencies, therapies, appointments and hopes all blurs into one. But at some point, she spent a long time on a haematology ward. Much to her dismay, she didn't have a private room this time. When I didn't need to be at my office, I'd sit by her bed, working on my laptop, occasionally taking the interminably slow lift down to the ground-floor shop to get her a newspaper or a drink. I came to recognise the patients in the other beds, by their faces for those well enough to be walking around, drip machines trundling along beside them, and by the tenor of their cries of pain or frustration for those who were sicker, hidden behind curtains or turned on their sides towards the walls. Some patients had lots of visitors; some had none. One young woman was visited most days by an older woman who wore a tunic similar to hospital scrubs over plain black trousers. She had an exhausted, harried manner. A backpack was slung over her shoulder and often half-unzipped as if she'd left somewhere in a rush. She'd sit beside the younger woman's bed, a few feet away from me, speaking inaudibly with her, then leave barely fifteen minutes later. One day, my mum wanted some Lucozade, so I happened to be waiting for that interminably slow lift at the same time as the harried woman. In London, it's conventional to ignore strangers, even if you're standing a foot away from them waiting for a lift. But in the parallel universe of the hospital, different rules apply, especially when you've seen someone around enough to know they're on a similar shitty journey to you. She told me that the young woman was her daughter, a sufferer of sickle cell anaemia.

'I come between shifts,' she said, 'when I can.'

I thought from her attire she was probably a care worker, so I asked and I was right. The lift came and I looked at our reflections in its mirror as we descended slowly through the hospital. We were the living embodiment of the story of women and care as it manifests in the twenty-first century. There was me, a white 'knowledge worker', middle class, able to be with my mother a lot, even if the juggle was a strain. And there was this lady beside me, leaning wearily against the handrail, a Black woman doing poorly paid shift work over which she probably had little to no control, taking care of someone else's family members while her own daughter suffered in hospital. We shared the sadness of watching a loved one in anguish, but our caregiving experience was completely different. Too often, narratives about care focus on one or other of these experiences. We need to witness both to create solutions that work for all women, not just some.

Coerced wives and daughters

In 1875, the wife of Thomas Grant filed a lawsuit in Iowa, USA. She'd cared for her husband 'during an insanity of sixteen months' prior to his death. A court had appointed her to perform this care, under the agreement that she'd be contractually entitled to $75 a month from his estate as recompense once he died. By the time she went to court, she believed she was due $1,500. On attempting to claim it, however, she was rejected. The judges' response to her suit dripped with sarcasm: 'Would the maintaining of an action against the husband for nursing him in sickness greatly promote the harmony of the marital relations or tend to increase domestic happiness and comfort?'[2]

Apparently, the idea of wives being compensated for caregiving was 'disastrous to the best interest of society'. They overruled the contract because caregiving was a service that 'she owed to her husband in virtue of the relation existing between them. She had no right to refuse to perform it, nor to demand compensation for performing it.' As Professor Glenn has explained in her book *Forced to Care: Coercion and Caregiving in America,* which details Mrs Grant's case and those of other women, if the story of care is a story of women, it's also a story of coercion. Debates rage about whether responsibility to provide care should be located in the family or in government, but whichever wins at each moment of history, thus far it has been women doing the actual tasks of caregiving.

The idea that caregiving ought to be a woman's role was not new to the nineteenth century, but it was crystallising in a very specific way around the time that Mrs Grant went to court. Before industrialisation, women had been productive members of their households, producing goods to be sold at market, like textiles, butter, cheese or eggs,[3] and ensuring the household had what it needed to run properly, for example by mending clothing or making candles. 'Home' and 'work' had been one and the same in this economy, which was organised around small-scale and subsistence agriculture. With industrialisation came new kinds of jobs and increasing urbanisation. This led to the separation of work and home, and with it, the separation of men and women into more clearly defined roles. The new woman would have been 'unrecognisable by her predecessor on the farm', write academics Enobong Hannah Branch and Melissa E. Wooten.[4] She was no longer an integral earner and producer within the family. Instead, men became the 'breadwinners', fighting to earn a 'family wage' that would be enough to keep themselves as well as a wife and children. Women were construed as being like children – as unproductive economic dependents, rather than as workers producing useful items and services for the family. Workers' unions in this period fought for higher wages to improve the lives of their families. No doubt this was laudable, but it also entrenched the ideal of a single, male breadwinner within a household, and in turn, women's economic dependency. Henry Broadhurst was a prominent nineteenth-century trade unionist and politician. In his 1877 speech to the annual conference of the umbrella body for trade unions in the UK, he told his fellow union members that they should 'as men and husbands . . . use their utmost efforts to bring about a condition of things, where their wives should be in their proper sphere at home, instead of being dragged into competition for livelihood against the great and strong men of the world'.[5]

Broadhurst and the Iowan judges presiding over Mrs Grant's case were advocating for the relatively new notion of the middle-class housewife, exemplified by the hugely popular mid-nineteenth-century poem 'The Angel in the House' by Coventry Patmore. Her *raison d'être* was to cultivate a comfortable and well-mannered home environment for her husband and children: 'Man must be pleased; but him to please /Is woman's pleasure.' According to Patmore, this ideal woman conducted herself with 'cloudless brow'. After all, a man needed a cosy hearth and worry-free home to return to after his hard day's labour, right? Women's lives, for those families that could afford it, became stories of infantilisation, dependency and domesticity.

It was predictable that proceedings wouldn't go in Mrs Grant's favour, given this context. But Martha Sullivan might have hoped for more. When she went to court in 1937, (white American women had been allowed to vote for seventeen years, after the Nineteenth Amendment was passed in 1920. Sullivan was a professional nurse, hired on a private contract by Andrew Sonnicksen to care for him. In return, she was to receive some of his property upon his death. While she was working for him, the nature of their relationship changed, and they married about eighteen months after she entered his employ. Then, upon his death, Martha discovered that Andrew hadn't left the agreed property to her in his will. The California Appeals Court saw no problem with this; because the pair had married, her services had transmuted into those freely provided by a wife, rendering the employment contract null and void. It wasn't deemed relevant that Martha had forgone considerable earnings as a professional to care for Andrew on the understanding of this future compensation. Instead, they felt that:

When the parties subsequently entered into a contract of marriage and became husband and wife, one of the implied terms of the contract of marriage was that appellant would perform without compensation the services covered by said written agreement . . . the necessary legal effect of the marriage contract as to terminate the obligations of the parties under said written agreement.[6]

In the hundred years since Martha Sullivan sought justice, the world has been remade many times over. We've had the advent of cars, the internet, the contraceptive pill and nuclear fission. We've discovered antibiotics and realised the harms of greenhouse gases for our ecosystem. We went to war in myriad new ways and built supranational bodies like the United Nations and NATO to try to protect peace. But for all our invention, discovery and geopolitical change, the idea that it's natural for women to want to provide care freely for loved ones – and that if they don't, there's something immoral about them – still holds. What would you think of me if I said I'd been reluctant to care for my mother? What would it mean about me as a woman? And how would that differ to hearing a man say the same?

'Everywhere, it is women,' Ulla tells me from her home in Kävlinge, southern Sweden, talking about caregiving around the world. Ulla and her husband are in their seventies and live near a small river, where she likes to walk and enjoy nature. Before we get into the nitty-gritty of her life as a caregiver, she tells me that she's been to the UK, where I live, because her father was a sea captain and took her on his boat across the North

Sea. Nowadays, her life is more stationary. One day, Ulla came home from work for lunch and saw her husband's legs on the floor in their bedroom, 'and then I understood something had happened'. As she recalls that day, the immediacy of it in her mind remains apparent, even years later. Today, her husband's brain is fine, but one arm and one leg don't function. Ulla is correct that most caregiving around the world is performed unpaid by women. This is true even in countries that are often referenced as exemplars of gender equality. In Ulla's homeland of Sweden, for example, more women are caregivers than men, and women who are caregivers are likely to provide more hours of help per week, and for more days of the week, than men who are caregivers.[7] This is despite the fact that the Nordic countries have made gender equality a priority for decades and now have amongst the highest female labour force participation rates in the Organisation for Economic Cooperation and Development (OECD) member countries.[8] They're a good example of what gender equality has come to mean: women work *and* care.

It's not only adult women who are affected by these norms; girls, too, are preferred over boys for unpaid caregiving. Anil Patil, the founder and executive director of Carers Worldwide whom we met in Chapter 1, told me that if a family member falls ill or has an accident in parts of southern India and no adult woman can provide care, it will probably mean a daughter will drop out of education to fulfil that role. In some cases, men abandon their families altogether when caring needs become apparent. Elineca Ndowo, whom we also met earlier, works with teachers in Tanzania to educate them in dealing with disabled children and reduce stigma. 'Not all – but many – men tend to separate with their wives when they have disabled children, meaning that first of all, they don't accept or they don't believe they can be the cause of the challenge. And others, they escape to avoid the responsibility of taking care, because it's sometimes consuming, financially expensive, and it's something which cannot end in the near time, so they normally escape.'[9] In general, she told me, around ninety per cent of the parent-care-givers she encounters are women. Patil and Ndowo are sharing experiences from the Global South and, while rigorous data on the same issue in the north is hard to find, anecdotes shared with me recount similar situations.

Helping versus caring

Even when men are involved in care, there are crucial differ-ences in the roles they undertake and the activities they perform compared to women. In general, if men perform care at all, it's more likely that they'll do so for their spouses than other people. They're also more likely to describe doing so out of love. In contrast, women are more likely to care for other relations too, such as elderly parents, and to describe doing so out of duty rather than love.[10] In most contemporary cultures, we have only one spouse, but we have many other relatives. This means that a woman's pool of potential caregiving is far larger than that of a man. When men *are* considered responsible for their elderly parents, this often manifests as financial responsibility rather than practical. It's their wives – so, the daughters-in-law of the people who need care – who perform the actual caregiving itself.

In September 2019, I arranged for my mother's siblings and paid professionals to cover me, caring for her while I went for a walk. An eleven-day walk. The Coast to Coast is a long-distance hiking trail from the west side of England to the east. The route goes through the world-famous beauty of the Lake District, which William Wordsworth described as 'the loveliest spot that man hath found'. From there, the terrain changes to bucolic farmland and then rolling moors, covered in purple heather and yellow gorse, until eventually, around 200 miles later, you reach the sea at the picturesque fishing village of Robin Hood's Bay. I walked it alone, seeking solitude. I met other people doing the same, mainly men of around retirement age. They were married, but their wives weren't with them. For some, it was because the women weren't interested in hiking. But a couple of them told me, without the slightest discomfort, that their wives couldn't join them because they needed to keep an eye on their elderly mothers. 'Their *own* mothers?' I clarified. No – the *husbands'* mothers. The mothers of the men out hiking this incredible trail, having the experience of a lifetime.

I grew up without a father present, and this lack of a template has led me to find the concept of fathers and husbands unfathomable at times. Interactions like those I had on the hiking trail, where the men were allegedly part of families but apparently living on their own terms at the expense of women, do nothing to clarify my confusion. Katy, whom we met in Chapter 1, told me of her brother: '[He] runs his own agricultural engineering business, so he's very busy all the time. He helps, he does help with . . . let's say my mum's shower isn't working, then he'll sort that out with me, so that sort of practical side of things that I don't know how to do.' Katy, meanwhile, does the day-to-day care for her mum, while also trying to care for her own husband. Karen's brother has taken on the role of financial management for their parents, which he performs at long distance while she does the continuous daily work of care. Both are exemplars of research findings that when sons participate in care, they're more likely to assume responsibility for tasks that aren't time-sensitive, whereas daughters will take on the day-to-day tasks that require consistent attention.[11]

Saints or whores: the dilemma of personal care

The idea that women were, and continue to be, uniquely suited to the domestic world rests uncomfortably alongside the bodily reality of caregiving. Patmore's ideal woman never frowned, yet the perfect woman of his era was also tending to the sick and the dying. She must have been either a psychopath or a Vulcan. In the very same period that women were meant to be floating elegantly around their hearths without a care in the world, the care they were actually administering would have meant encountering pneumonia, typhus, typhoid fever, diphtheria, scarlet fever, measles, whooping cough, dysentery and tuber-culosis.[12] Halloween provides a surprising manifestation of this contradiction between the pure and the bodily, the perfect and the diseased. Head to a costume party, and you're likely to find a few 'sexy nurses' in attendance. This stereotype is centuries old: in medieval Europe, single women who tended to the sick but weren't nuns were often accused of being licentious and of selling sex.[13] After all, they visited men alone, and sometimes at night. They tended to these men's bodies, washing them, and who knew what else . . . Dr Christa Wichterich, a sociologist at the University of Basel, has described how women working as nurses in India have been subject to the same misogynist mores:

> . . .prejudices regarding the morality of nurses emerged because earlier they often stayed unmarried, having to take care of male patients and do nightshift . . . Today, the image of nurses as care workers is caught up in the dilemma between care ethics and loose morals, nobleness and impurity, saint and whore.[14]

Women have been defined as the most appropriate of our species to provide care, yet also judged as being morally impure for the proximity to nakedness that care requires. And while those ideas about moral impurity have largely died out, still it remains women who are invariably deployed to perform intimate care, such as bathing people and changing incontinence wear. If you haven't been a caregiver, you might think this aspect applies only to a minority of people needing care. I'd probably have thought that before my mum got sick. But in reality, many people, of all ages and with all sorts of impairments, need support with washing and going to the toilet. Very old people and those with certain conditions, such as Parkinson's or motor neurone diseases, along with those who've had ravaging cancer treatments like my mum, often become incontinent. This includes urinary and bowel incontinence. It's shockingly common, yet almost entirely unspoken about. It's hard to gauge the precise scale because people don't report it or aren't asked about it, but we can assess it by the size of the adult incontinence product market. In 2020, the global market value reached US $15.4 billion and is projected to hit US $24.2 billion by 2026.[15] The demand for these products for over sixty-fives now outstrips that of those for infants.[16] It's astonishing, really, that something so prevalent and so likely to be part of our own lives, both as caregivers and as we age, is unknown beyond the bounds of care and medicine. And given the scale, it's obvious that unless we change our assumptions about women being more appropriate to perform intimate tasks, we're never going to solve the gender inequality of care.

Ayesha is thirty-three and lives in Kathmandu, Nepal. She is compassionate and articulate throughout our conversation, and certainly wise beyond her years, which is unsurprising given what she's been through. At the time of her mother's cancer diagnosis, she owned a restaurant with a man who was also her romantic partner. I found her through a mutual contact based in Kenya, marvelling at the power of twenty-first-century technology to connect me so easily with different time zones and countries. 'My granddad or my brother or any of the men who were present in the room would always leave,' she explains to me when I ask about how intimate tasks were performed for her mother. 'So intimacy is okay when it's shared with women. But I think when men are involved, it just becomes very complicated, because shame looks very different in front of a man.'

Kathmandu and London are 5,415 miles apart, yet while Ayesha was navigating these social mores in her city, I was doing the same in mine. My mother had a sister and brother still alive at the time of her death. Both came to help in stints during her illness, for which I was immensely grateful. Towards the end of her life, my mother could no longer walk or move much at all. She lay in a white metal hospital bed that had been moved into her bedroom, and her bedside table was scattered with pill boxes and barely sipped nutritional drinks. She had taken on the look of the dying: simultaneously puffy and withering. Because she couldn't get out of bed, and because she was also suffering from bowel incontinence due to her cancer treatments, she needed changing frequently. The scene I'm describing was harrowing emotionally and hard work physically. She could just about move her hips, but doing so was uncomfortable for her and she often seemed confused or irritated by the request. Every time I asked her to move, coaxing and soothing her, I was having to hurt and anger her to make her clean. The need to seek permission for a man – my uncle, her brother – to learn to change her so that, if need be, he could be left alone with her, was an additional burden. It wasn't his fault; he was totally willing and unfailingly helpful. The point is rather that there you are, in the hardest situation of your life, and there's suddenly an obstacle thrown into your path, an uncomfortable topic to be broached on top of everything else that's happening. Who is allowed to perform intimate care? What's your mum comfortable with? Is she only saying she's comfortable with it because she can hear the desperate exhaustion in your voice? What does dignity mean to her? And for the man in question – is he OK with this strange breach of gender protocol? Are you imposing by asking for it, even though it was imposed on you with no one asking? When did your life change so thoroughly that this is the stuff of your days? Like all of caregiving, it's a collective problem obscured because it plays out in individual bedrooms around the world. And it's a topic people would rather avoid altogether. Raise the increasing rate of bowel incontinence to the people you encounter over the next few days and watch them freak out and scuttle past it – trust me, I've tried. But without addressing this aspect of care, we can't move forward. What equality can be achieved if you, or someone you love, is going to prefer one gender over another to provide their intimate care?

When we dodge these conversations, we play directly into the 'angel in the house' stereotype, in which 'life is sweetest when it's clean'.[17] Caring for people is too often conceptualised as 'nice', but it involves some of the hardest tasks. Breaking bodies fall apart in every way imaginable – and several ways that are not until they're in front of you. You'll be cleaning sores, pushing emollient cream into hitherto private crevices, changing incontinence pads, mopping up vomit and washing dried-out skin. It's not 'feminine' in the sense that we understand that word. And so, when we decide that only women can be present and comfortable with nakedness and its attendant vulnerability, we also decide that women will do the majority of care for our species.

Free does not mean without cost

Using women as the caregivers of our species has been construed as natural and, consequently, women have cared for free. However, free does not mean without cost. The history of women overflows with stories of jobs left and careers abandoned because of the obligation to perform care. I did exactly this in 2020, leaving my job and its associated career path in order to be with my mum in the final months of her life. My resignation was more of a choice than that of many historical women, because I could have tried to take compassionate leave from work, or refused to look after my mum. But as much as those were possibilities in theory, in practice it didn't feel like they were. Taking leave from work for an extended and indefinite period (you can't predict how quickly someone will die) isn't conventional. Nor did I want to keep working and for my mum to be with strangers in her last weeks. In this way, the only real difference between me and the many generations of women caregivers before me was our clothing style. Take Mrs Andrews, a teacher in the late-nineteenth century. In 1897, the School Board was considering firing her because she'd failed to legitimise her many absences. Her husband wrote to them and explained that this was due to 'the illness and death of my father, her father and mother, and five of our children'.[18] Poor Mrs Andrews had been caring for eight people; those gaps in her CV, like mine, were muted tales of arduous bodily toil and bereavement. We don't know what Mrs Andrews thought about this, but her contemporary, Jane Addams, was angry. Addams wanted a medical career, but had to forgo it in order to care for her mentally unwell older brother. In 1915, some years after this life path was thrust upon her, Addams published an essay entitled 'Filial Relations', in which she railed at her parents' failure to respect her career dreams and to recognise them as a 'genuine and dignified claim'.[19]

Addams clearly felt robbed of the life she'd wanted, coerced into caregiving against her will. She's one of many, in her own era and today, in her native USA and all over the world. Ayesha was studying ecological economics at university in Nepal when her father fell ill. She left her degree to help her mother care for him, intending to return and complete it after he died. Then her mother became sick. Ayesha never went back to her studies. 'Did it impact my life? Absolutely,' she tells me. 'I mean, I was supposed to go back to university, which I didn't when my dad was ill, and it's just been one thing after the other. So all of my life plans towards what I wanted my career to be and what I had kind of aspired [to], I had to change that pretty fast, I would say.'

Josie lives in Cornwall, a coastal area in the southwest of England that is beloved for its beauty, both rugged and picturesque. She cares for her son, who has Asperger's, dyspraxia and ADHD. When he was born, she was studying psychology and hoped to become a forensic psychologist. Twenty-two years later, she's working in the cleaning industry because it's flexible enough to fit around her caring responsibilities. Reducing women's ability to work also means reducing their income. We heard in Chapter 1 how Katy and Karen's finances have been harmed by caregiving. Josie feels the same, describing constant hardship:

Oh, it's been such a struggle . . . It's just scraping together every week. You go shopping and you've got to buy [meals] for your family for the week, and you've just really got to be so careful what you pick. You can't just go for what you want to eat. You're on a really tight budget. You've got to add it up as you go along. Then you're left, sometimes [for] days, with nothing, nothing at all in the bank. [You] don't have any savings. There's nothing in the bank. You're just scraping by.

She's had to use food banks some weeks to ensure no one is going hungry. She's far from alone.

The hidden toll of caregiving on women's lives is all-pervading, affecting everything from income to sense of identity, from social lives to dreams. The research proves it, but every caregiver, including me, knows it because we've lived it. It begs the question: what is a woman if she exists only to meet someone else's needs? Is it right that the shape of someone's life is decided based on their gender, instead of anything about them as a person, their skills, aptitudes or interests? Consider this thought experiment: at some point in your life (most likely, but not necessarily, during your middle age), whatever job you've been doing, whatever passion you've been pursuing, whatever future you've envisaged, you will suddenly be given no choice but to resign, stop and be enrolled in an indefinite contract doing work that has nothing in common with those previous jobs or passions. Oh, and you won't be paid for it. Nor will you be recognised or respected. You'll work long and exhausting hours, with some elements that cause you back pain, wrist pain, sleep deprivation. You will have no control over any of your work's components. And no, you'll have no right to complain. In fact, there isn't even a boss to complain to.

How do you feel about that? Welcome to the history and the present of the majority of women around the world.

Wages for Housework and the parent–child problem

It's striking and sad that things remain this way, because in the 1970s, the 'Wages for Housework' campaign attempted to change this situation of oppression and inequality. The idea that women could be defined outside their own control and have their lives relegated to domestic drudgery was violently rejected. Women came together in countries as far apart as the UK and Mexico to demand liberation from patriarchy and more autonomy over their lives. The call of 'wages for housework' was a central part of this movement. This could be understood as both a literal demand – pay us for all the hours we put into domestic labours – and also as a tactic to shift how housework and childcare were understood. Were these activities 'unproductive' in comparison with the men's factory work? The movement challenged the dominant discourse, arguing that domestic labours were indeed *labours* – after all, raising the next generation of workers and feeding the current one were hardly tasks society could cope without. The campaigners used the term 'reproductive labour' to capture the importance of what women did in the home; they were reproducing the very basis of life on which the 'productive' workforce relied. Wages for Housework called for this change in understanding and, along with it, an end to women's remuneration in 'the coin of "love" and "virtue"', as political theorist Nancy Fraser has described it, instead of real money.[20] The movement challenged the sexist reasoning we saw earlier from the judges in the cases of Mrs Grant and Martha Sullivan, and it challenged the very basis on which much of our legal, political and economic systems were built.

Along with this attempt at re-categorising domestic labours, solutions were put forward to reduce the volume and intensity of those labours. Chief amongst these solutions was that domestic tasks should be aggregated and performed at a collective level. Nurseries are a version of this – a handful of adults can care for many children at once, rather than each child being cared for by an individual – and probably isolated – woman. This approach shifts care out of the private domestic sphere and into the public shared sphere. It can reduce isolation, workload and costs. 'Childcare should be socialised, meal preparation should be socialised, housework should be industrialised . . .' wrote political activist and professor Angela Davis in her seminal 1981 book, *Women, Race and Class*.[21]

Interventions like this can work well. 'Meals on wheels is a great thing!' Tracy tells me from Michigan. They deliver meals to her father three days a week, reducing the amount of time she spends supporting him, which is generally between two and six hours each day (without any predictability as to which day will require which length of time). Respite and day centres for people who need care and those who support them can be invaluable, providing a space to socialise, pursue passions and seek advice, or have time off caregiving. Carers Worldwide has initiated twenty-five community caring centres in India, Nepal and Bangladesh. At these centres, two paid care workers support those with extra needs, enabling the family caregivers to be elsewhere. For adults, this is likely to mean they can work to earn money. Sometimes, the family caregiver is a child, and having these centres means they can go to school. Before this initiative, all these people were caring individually. Now two paid workers can care for many people at once, and families are better off because there's more household income. Line lives in Norway, a country with a global reputation for socialised services. Although she's keen to impress upon me that all is not perfect there, it's evident that the array of free services for her son, including a day centre and one week per month of respite care, has meant she can stay in her career as a music teacher and musician, an aspect of her life that brings her great satisfaction. It's a relief to find a caregiver who's been able to carry on with their passion in amongst the many stories of loss after loss.

However, the scale of change imagined by the second-wave feminists has not materialised. This would have required changes not just to the organisation of our domestic lives, but also to the very foundations on which the modern welfare state was built. In 1942, British civil servant William Beveridge published a report that outlined how a government of the future should care for its citizens. It would, he said, provide a minimum standard of living from cradle to grave, and tackle the 'five giants' of Want, Disease, Ignorance, Squalor and Idleness. But Beveridge had a blind spot: sexism. In an earlier book on unemployment, he wrote that the 'ideal unit is the household of man, wife and children maintained by the earnings of the first alone'.[22] He recognised the importance of domestic activities, saying that 'the great majority of married women must be regarded as occupied on work which is vital though unpaid, without which their husbands could not do their paid work and without which the nation could not continue',[23] but seemed to view that 'vital work' as a natural expression of femininity, rather than something a woman might not wish to do, something a man might do instead, or for which a woman might wish to be paid. Consequently, caregivers were not included within Beveridge's era-defining report.

Attempting to win feminist demands under the rubric of the welfare state was like trying to fit a square peg into a round hole. As an example, consider a supposed success of the welfare state in 1975. The British government introduced the Invalid Care Allowance, a benefit available to people who provided regular care to a severely disabled relative, and a precursor of the 'Carer's Allowance' we have in the UK today.[24] Robert Boscawen, a politician for a well-to-do constituency in south-west England, described the merits of this new policy:

> It is a small innovation in terms of cash, but it does something that has long been needed for a very small group of people— namely, those devoted daughters and nieces, and friends we hope, who have looked after a parent or a disabled relative over many years at great cost and even hardship to themselves.[25]

Of course, he didn't mention sons and nephews alongside daughters and nieces. More importantly, the allowance was payable to men who'd given up paid employment to care for somebody, and to *single* women who'd had to do the same. Married or cohabiting women? No. They were ineligible for the benefit because of their assumed economic dependency on the men in their lives.[26] It was exactly 100 years since Mrs Grant had stood in the dock in Iowa asking for her contractually agreed payment, yet the same reasoning remained. As political theorist Professor Carole Pateman has described it: 'Welfare state policies have ensured in various ways that wives/women provide welfare services gratis, disguised as part of their responsibility for the private sphere.' In the USA, academics have described the welfare state as 'two-tiered', with men receiving benefits as workers and women receiving them on a secondary basis as dependents of the men.[27]

If you spend time reading documents from second-wave feminism, caregiving of the type with which we're concerned is conspicuously absent. Most care-related concerns focused on motherhood and conventional childcare. In August 1970, 50,000 women marched down New York's Fifth Avenue carrying signs that included the slogans 'Free Universal Childcare' and 'Free Abortion on Demand'.[28] In Mexico, the Feminist Women's Coalition campaigned for 'voluntary motherhood'. They wanted sex education, reliable and inexpensive contraceptives, abortion rights, and an end to forced sterilisations. The four demands of the UK's incipient Women's Liberation Movement were announced in 1971: equal pay, equal educational and job opportunities, free contraception and abortion on demand, and free twenty-four-hour nurseries.[29] The parent–child relationship was the focus, and remains the paradigmatic care relationship today; all others are understood with reference to it. This became hugely frustrating to me during my time as a caregiver, and today I'm still continuously conscious of how often people's assumptions and language imply that 'parent–child' is the only caring relationship within families that is exhausting, demanding and in need of support. A list shared online titled 'You know you're a mom when . . .' includes 'you fantasise about sleeping' and 'cleaning up is a pointless exercise': experiences that are equally applicable to caregivers, but they're not part of our social discussion. The omission of caregivers from our awareness means that many feminist demands only work for parenting, and not for the kind of caregiving with which we're concerned here. For the parent–child dyad, collective forms of care, like nurseries or after-school centres, make sense as proposed solutions because we presume parents have rightful power over their children's lives. They impose that power when they send their kid to those places, freeing themselves up for work or other pursuits. But what about when you're talking about *adults who need care,* not kids? Is it acceptable to impose such choices upon them? Consider yourself: what will you want when you're old and infirm? Will you appreciate being dropped off somewhere every day with people of differing ages, belief systems and impairments, with whom who haven't chosen to spend time? It can work really well for some people – the users of the centres in Nepal and Bangladesh initiated by Carers Worldwide are a good example – but we certainly shouldn't presume that all elderly and impaired people will be keen on this kind of option. When my mum was well enough to go to a day centre, there's no way in hell she'd have agreed if I'd suggested it, and when she was sicker, there's no way in hell I'd have tried to send her somewhere that might not be set up for her complex and unpredictable needs, which changed from week to week.

Carlyle and Barb live in Minneapolis. Barb had a stroke in

March 2017 and is now wheelchair-bound with chronic pain that 'goes from zero to nine just instantly'. She is also aphasic; she can communicate but can't pronounce words in a conventional way. And she's obsessed with Diet Coke. Carlyle is her husband, a charismatic man in his mid-seventies and the recipient of a prestigious US prize for playwrights. In 2020, he wrote a new play about what he and Barb have been through, describing the experience of her stroke and their subsequent and radically altered life together. He laughs as he tells me that part of the reason he's OK with their situation now, as hard as it can be at times, is that in his 'younger life, I just spent that youth to death'. Barb sits beside him with an open and expressive face. Even though the sounds she makes lack precise forms or consonants to turn them into full words, I find I can still understand much of what she wants to convey from the glint in her eyes, by turns mischievous, frustrated or agreeable.

When Barb first got out of hospital after her stroke, she stayed in a rehabilitation centre. 'We got asked to leave,' Carlyle tells me. 'We got thrown out because she was a flight risk. She kept going outside in the street, going across the street [to] the park. One time, they found her in a grocery store.' As he recounts this, Barb is looking less than impressed. She'd been in that grocery store, Carlyle explains, because she'd wanted some of her beloved 'pop' to drink, and also to regain some sense of independence. Her mission was unlikely to succeed because she couldn't speak and had no money, but I think we can all understand the impulse. However, because she's disabled, and regardless of the fact that anyone of us might do the same, her errand was considered a breach of the rules. 'They didn't seem to be making any provision for the fact that Barb's a human being,' Carlyle says.

I tell them that it reminds me of the story of Nellie Bly, the pioneering nineteenth-century journalist who posed as mentally unwell and had herself committed to a New York City asylum to expose its dire conditions. Once inside, her protestations of sanity fell on deaf ears and she was only released when the newspaper for which she worked took it up with the asylum. She recounted:

> I said to one [doctor], 'You have no right to keep sane people here. I am sane, have always been so and I must insist on a thorough examination or be released. Several of the women here are also sane. Why can't they be free?'
>
> 'They are insane,' was the reply, 'and suffering from delusions.'[30]

Once Bly was labelled as 'abnormal', her own words or needs were irrelevant. 'Oh, yes,' Barb says when I recount this, nodding vigorously. 'Oh yes.'

Aside from the important issue of people's choices about how and where they're cared for, there's a deeper problem with the idea that we can meet caregiving needs while still liberating ourselves from them. The need for care doesn't disappear; the 'devoted daughter or niece' might be liberated, but who takes on the role of caregiver instead?

Other women.

From slave to migrant care worker

When we embarked on this chapter, I said there are two categories of women when it comes to caregiving. We've met the first, our Snow Whites who allegedly adore taking care of all those around them, have little purpose outside of other people's needs and are fulfilled by drudgery. Now let's meet the second category. Unlike the wives and daughters we've met so far, who were caring for family members, here we meet the women who are caring for people because it's their paid work, like the lady with whom I shared that slow lift down through hospital on my mission to buy Lucozade. Although in this book we're predominantly concerned with kin caregivers, not paid care workers, we still need to spend a bit of time exploring the latter to see where we've gone so wrong with care overall.

Before the early twentieth century and the abolition of chattel slavery, the women who spent their lives caring for other people's families without the option of caring for their own weren't paid care workers at all, but enslaved people. Like paid care workers today, enslaved women could only care for their families when they weren't required to work, and that work included caring for their masters' sick or elderly family members.[31] After abolition, enslaved people were replaced with domestic servants, who weren't legally owned by their employers but were still subject to harsh and often exploitative conditions. Domestic servants still exist today, now often termed 'domestic workers'. And aside from live-in domestic workers, nowadays we also have paid care workers, who work either in institutions like care homes or in private houses.

In the USA today, women of colour comprise over half of all care workers.[32] This is substantially more than is proportionate within the population, which is around twenty-eight per cent non-white overall. The roots of this bias can be traced back to post-slavery regulations.[33] Not all jobs were open to Black women after abolition – domestic work was one of the few occupations available to them until the 1960s.[34] Black women were also preferred in such roles because they were viewed as more submissive. An 1872 article in the *New York Times* explained why Americans of African descent made 'excellent' servants:

> They do not have to learn to keep their 'places' . . . In the not universal quality of kindness to children, they are simply excellent by the laws of their gentle, cheerful, grateful natures. They are the coming help, the servants of the future . . . These colored people, for the present at least, have acquired few of the vices of the superior race of servants . . . and they are so unconscious of the indignity of fully earning their wages that they are likely to do twice the work of other kinds of servants without regarding themselves overtaxed.[35]

During season seven of hit American TV show *The Big Bang Theory*, Mrs Wolowitz – the mother of main character Howard Wolowitz – breaks her leg and requires care. The season includes several episodes poking fun at the impaired old lady and her needs, with none of her loved ones wanting to support her. At one point, her son Howard says he and his wife should 'get a nurse; preferably someone from a third-world country who's used to suffering and unpleasant smells'.[36] There's tinny laughter from the live studio audience. The script is in extremely poor taste, but it's nonetheless accurate about the likely origin of care workers today: they're not only likely to be non-white, but also to be migrants from poorer countries than those in which they work. Over twenty per cent of healthcare support workers in the USA are migrants.[37] Across Europe, too, it's usual to find care sectors disproportionately dominated by migrants from poorer countries. Much of this is shaped by former colonial histories, such as in Italy, where it's been common for care workers to be migrants from its former colonies of Somalia, Ethiopia, Eritrea, Cape Verde and the Philippines.[38]

The choice to become a care worker upon migrating is based on a range of constraints and assumptions. Qualifications are often unrecognised between countries, so migrants must go into work that doesn't require them. Because caregiving has been devalued as 'women's work' for so long, in many countries it's a sector with very low barriers to entry. Singapore provides a useful example: the process involved in registration of foreign nurses and midwives is complex, and often results in foreign nurses having to downgrade, for example from a nurse to a nursing aide, if they do not meet the criteria.[39] Care that involves living in someone's home can also be especially attractive for migrants compared to other low-waged work, as it provides both work and shelter. And when we factor in the stereotyping of women as natural caregivers, and of specific racialised groups as more 'appropriate' for care work, it makes sense that many migrant women either choose care work or end up finding it the only available option. Academics have labelled this pattern 'care extractivism', showing how the removal of caring capacity from poorer countries leaves those countries depleted in this essential human resource.[40] This creates 'global care chains', as people in wealthier countries use migrants from poorer places to provide care.[41] In turn, the children or elderly parents of those migrant care workers are left missing a crucial part of their own care network, and someone from a poorer family in that origin country is hired to step in – and on it goes.

It's a horrible thought, that the story of caregiving in the twenty-first century has become one of direct exploitation between women across continents. Although this is partly a product of globalisation, it is in fact the reconfiguration of the long-standing arrangement between the powerful and the powerless that travels over time, from enslaved person to domestic servant to care worker. There is a deep and painful irony to acknowledge here: the liberation of one category of women has been at the cost of others' freedoms and choices, leaving them relegated to that very burdensome, undervalued toil, and preventing them from caring for their own sick loved ones. It's the kind of uncomfortable truth that my mother's generation of feminists might not have noticed or thought about, partly because globalisation was less developed when they were making their demands for liberation, and perhaps also partly because they were too desperate to be relieved of carrying care for our species. But today, with anti-racist politics becoming increasingly mainstream and the global media reporting on places far from our own homes, we can't ignore the impact of our choices.

When Jojo Moyes' bestselling novel *Me Before You* was made into a film in 2016, one promotional blurb read: 'After becoming unemployed, Louisa Clark is forced to accept [a job] which requires her to take care of Will Traynor, a paralysed man.'[42] Care work is, then, an unattractive option, something that Louisa is 'forced' to accept because of her misfortunes. Louisa has rather a good time, as it turns out, as she and Will fall in love (until he flies to Dignitas to end his life). But in general, it's true that paid care work is a bad option. For a start, it's appallingly paid, despite being such a vital job. In the UK, around half of professional care workers are paid less than a living wage, while in the US, award-winning investigative journalism has exposed severe exploitation in the sector, finding workers earning $2 an hour and suffering 'rampant wage theft', sleep deprivation and no time off.[43] Shockingly, one sixth of home care workers live below the federal poverty line.[44]

If a care worker is employed casually by an individual or their family, their working conditions will be subject to the whims of those people. This can work well: perhaps the employer is respectful of the care worker's time and needs, and provides paid sick leave and holiday. For many live-in care workers, unfortunately, this isn't the case. According to Dr Christa Wichterich, the increasing trend to have twenty-four-hour live-in care workers for the elderly in Western Europe is a 'semi-feudal form of care work', with workers underpaid and expected to be available constantly.[45] Alternatively, if you're employed by an agency or government service, you may be on a precarious contract, have shift times that are too short to allow you to perform tasks adequately, be unpaid for travel time between those shifts, and have limited or no rights or benefits. You'll also be expected to treat your care work as if you were on a factory production line, performing your tasks in neat, measurable and 'efficient' ways that are closely monitored. New technologies are exacerbating this. On 13 December 2016, US President Barack Obama signed the 21st Century Cures Act into law. Part of this Act required states to introduce 'electronic visit verification' (EVV) systems for Medicaid-funded personal care services. EVV apps track care workers, including their location, the time spent at each place, and the tasks performed. Roll-outs have been disastrous for several reasons, including technical glitches leaving care workers out of pocket by hundreds of dollars in a month.[46] The inclusion of 'geo-fencing' is also causing problems. This sets a maximum distance around a client's home that a care worker is allowed to travel without being flagged as 'non-compliant', preventing clients and their care workers from running errands, visiting family or friends, and carrying out similar activities.[47] Inevitably, this will mean kin caregivers have even more to do than before.

Even if geo-fencing was removed and glitches were fixed, EVV and similar methods by which care workers are tracked and surveilled leave no room for the fundamental unpredictability of care. In Chapter 1, I described the 'bodily reality of care' – a recognition of the fact that sick bodies cannot be expected to stick to a routine or remain the same from one week to the next. It may be feasible to build a routine around people with impairments that are relatively stable, but flux is always possible. It may take five minutes one morning to help someone to the toilet; it may take fifty-five the next. Anyone who's been a caregiver knows this. And when we compress the time available to perform care, measure it according to 'efficiency' and try to standardise it, we harm the quality of care and also push out the relational and emotional aspects – those aspects that we may well consider to be inextricable from its very concept. One woman, interviewed by researchers for the University of Leeds, UK, described her experience of trying to arrange paid care for her father:

> He has one very, very good carer ... he thinks the world of him ... But he has every Thursday off, every other weekend off, and he goes on holiday a lot ... I said [to the organisation providing the care workers], 'Can we have the same carers come in, he gets familiar with them, they get familiar with him,' and she said, 'We can't do that – they become too familiar with their clients.'[48]

It's a problem, then, to become 'familiar' with someone for whom you perform intimate tasks, according to today's care industry. The care worker shuttles between patients all day, becoming the embodiment of a conflict between our human understanding of 'care' and the market logic that's penetrated its provision. As Dr Wichterich describes it: 'The actual conflict between the logic of caring and the logic of profit-making is downloaded to the individual person, who has to manage time constraints, bureaucratic requirements of standardisation and documentation and their inner conflicts between efficiency and emotional bonds.'[49] This inevitably puts more pressure on family caregivers, because they're the only person able to fulfil the emotional needs of the person who requires support, let alone step in and fill the gaps left by too-short shifts.

Alternatives to this rationalistic and economising (or arguably, miserly) approach to the care industry do exist. The Equal Care Co-op is lauded as a new way forward. Based in the UK and still very young, it describes itself as 'facilitating caregiving relationships'.[50] It's co-owned and run by its members, who comprise clients of care services, their kin caregivers, care workers, and investors. This is an example of what's known as 'stakeholder' ownership – everyone who has a stake in an entity has a say. Contrast this with care services provided by the private sector, which are governed by owners seeking to make profits, or those run by governments with faceless bureaucrats and maze-like systems, where little consideration may be given as to how decisions will affect people's lives.

Adelola and me

By autumn 2019, I'd already spent a couple of years trying to do everything at once, and I was exhausted to the point of blacking out one morning on my daily commute to work. With my mum's permission, I sought paid care workers so that I would have some small periods of time each week when I knew I only needed to worry about doing my job. Having spent several years working on social justice campaigns, my first question when I rang round local care companies was about the working conditions and pay of their staff. The manager of the first company I called told me, 'Oh, they'll always say they're not getting enough, but just ignore them. It's better than they'd get back home, anyway.' Thankfully, I found an ethical company shortly after, one that paid its workers a proper living wage and had a minimum shift time of two hours, meaning both my mum and the workers could feel unhurried as they did whatever was needed. But not everyone lives in an area with ethical care companies or has the funds to pay for them, and the lack of availability of good quality care takes a toll on kin caregivers. I know this all too well.

The night before my mother died, a healthcare assistant called Adelola from a local government-funded charity came to the house to sit up with me, a service available if you're at home with a dying person. It was invaluable to have her there, even though she was a stranger. It helped to blunt the lancing loneliness of being by myself beside my dying mother, sitting through the dark night as I watched her fight her imminent departure. When Adelola arrived, she and I chatted in the kitchen as she filled up her hot water bottle from the kettle. She was used to working night shifts, and she knew what made her feel comfortable and helped her get through the long vigil. She seemed tired, and I asked if she'd been working the night before too. Yes, she said. She paused and then her shoulders deflated. She told me she'd spent the early hours of that very morning with a woman in her early thirties who'd died. The woman's husband and their young children had been there too. Adelola teared up. 'It doesn't normally get to me because it's my job, but she was so young, and her babies were there,' she explained, screwing on the top of her hot water bottle and looking down at the kitchen countertop. I said she must have wished she had tonight off. She said she was supposed to, but they were understaffed. I apologised, told her to leave early if she wanted, that I'd cope. My mother was dying upstairs, and yet because of the system we've created, I was worrying about the wellbeing of the woman sent to support me.

Like me and the woman in the lift, here I was beside Adelola faced once again with the stark reality that our care system is divided by economic class, migration status and race. Throughout my time as a caregiver, I was repeatedly told how 'strong' I was. But Adelola, a Black migrant working-class woman, is expected to bear any burden her poorly paid work places upon her. The way that we, as a species, have arranged care is not working for kin caregivers nor paid care workers. In the Snow White version of care, its reality – bodily, arduous, exhausting, costly in all the ways we've seen – is overlooked, and care is seen as a function of love and kindness, a joy for the woman serving this natural capability. Thus, as with Mrs Grant and the married women who might have wanted access to the Invalid C Allowance, care is *valorised* but not *valued,* as academic Emma Dowling has described it.[51] And this failure to value caregiving in the home translates in the job market into one of the worst jobs around. Here, care is recognised as hard physical work, but its value is purely monetary – a question of efficiency and productivity in accordance with market logic.

One commonly deployed solution is to try to relabel care as 'work', as we saw with the 1970s feminist movement. 'Care work is work' remains a popular political slogan, wherein the word 'care' is used to encompass all forms of care, including parenting, kin caregiving and poorly paid care work. In dictionary definition terms, 'work' means the performance of a task or set of tasks for a particular purpose, or some variation on that theme, whether paid or not. Most human activities, then, could be called 'work' if we apply the term widely. It can be something you find meaningful, like me writing this book, or something that is pure and unpleasant toil, like cleaning toilets in strangers' houses. There are some immediate problems with defining caregiving in this way. If caregiving is work, then what about young caregivers – that is, kids who are caregiving for siblings or parents with impairments? In Kenya, where there's been an attempt to eradicate 'child labour', this has caused problems, with child caregivers being deemed child labourers. This has led to child caregivers lacking support because the authorities fear being seen to support child labour.[52] Putting caregiving into the category of work is useful for highlighting its arduous nature; the long hours, the lack of breaks, the tasks like lifting that can cause physical harm. In the work world, we legislate and regulate for those things and we picket our employers. How do we picket love? The tools we need are different to those we imagine when we think in terms of work. Finally, it implies that solving the problem of care is as simple as paying caregivers (and paying paid care workers properly), which it isn't, as we'll see throughout these pages.

Really, defining care as 'work' is a tactic to try to get care properly valued. Under capitalism, paid work (understood as productive, taking place in the market and with a historical bias towards men) is a far more valued kind of activity than care (understood as unproductive, taking place in the private home and with a historical bias towards women). This is evident in the origins of the welfare state, as we've seen. Wouldn't it be helpful if care could also be seen as work, and therefore socially valued and worthy of remuneration and respect? It would certainly go a long way towards righting the wrongs occurring, but it's far from a whole solution. Instead, we must interrogate why 'work' is the only category of activity that gets to be on a pedestal. Some activists and thinkers believe the real purpose of calls like 'wages for housework' is just that – by exposing the invisible labour of care and domestic work, we can create a rupture in our economic arrangements, forcing a better future for everyone. As feminist theorist Sophie Lewis explained in her 2019 book, *Full Surrogacy Now: Feminism against Family,* calling for wages for feminised work 'is not a petition, and it does not describe an exciting destination . . . it describes a process of assault on wage society'.[53] Unfortunately, as she also notes, the call has a tendency to be watered down and turned into bureaucratic exercises that may tot up the hours of unpaid, invisible work we do, but fail to challenge our economic system and underlying attitudes towards gender as a whole.

An alternative, and potentially more effective, way of thinking about caregiving is given to us by feminist theorists Joan Tronto and Berenice Fisher. They describe it as 'a species activity that includes everything that we do to maintain, continue and repair our "world" so that we can live in it as well as possible'.[54] In terms of caregiving for the sick, impaired and elderly, the content of that activity changes depending on the era and culture. It's not actually 'natural', per se, to care for those who are unable to care for themselves. Practices of infanticide and senicide aren't unknown. But care has become the moral convention, one of which I'm sure many of us are glad. If then, caregiving is a species activity – an essential component of being human and of human life in the way we live now – then it shouldn't need to be relabelled and redefined as 'work' in order to be valued sufficiently. Having a job, in the current economic arrangements of most of the world, is an essential part of life. Caregiving, in the current cultural arrangements of most of the world, is essential too. They stand shoulder to shoulder as things we should expect from our lives as humans, here and now, rather than one being stacked above the other. And recognising caregiving as important in its own right pushes back against the tendency to treat it as either an addendum to 'real work' or as a rare experience.

Think about it: if we're lucky enough to live into old age, we're likely to become impaired. We don't often describe the infirm elderly as 'disabled', but they are. Their impairments – not being able to walk much, needing wheelchair accessibility, their hands not having the dexterity to type or punch in telephone numbers, and so on – do not match up with the way the world works, turning these impairments into 'disabilities'. If we're all on the path towards disabilities, whether through accident, illness or old age, it's absurd to treat caregiving as a surprise, a problem, or, indeed, as an economic sector. It's a natural fact of existence, like breathing. This is also why we keep turning away from resolving the problems of caregiving as they are today: to understand caregiving as an inescapable part of life means acknowledging our own vulnerabilities. We want to 'continue the myth of our own invulnerable autonomy', writes Tronto. So we ignore caregiving issues unless they collide with our own lives, and we describe the whole thing as a 'burden'. Etymologically, 'burden' comes from the Old English *byrðen*, which has an interesting dual meaning. Expectedly, it means 'a load, weight, charge, duty', but it also means 'a child', i.e. that which is borne. We conceive of care as a load we carry, and we lack other ways of understanding it that aren't negative or don't rely on the paradigm of parent–child. No wonder so much mental strain is experienced by caregivers. They inhabit a parallel dimension that the well world tries not to see. Describing care as work doesn't overcome this problem. It redesignates it as something of value, but still keeps it neatly and comfortably cordoned off from what it means to be human. I didn't need to be told that I was a 'worker' when I was caring for my mum. I needed to be seen exactly as I was, and for that to be enough.

Make everyone a woman

We must move past solutions that rely on women in the home or women in the paid care sector – both treat us as a sub-class of human beings. What we need is a new gender logic; otherwise, we'll perpetuate the current sexism of our caring arrangements. Writing this, I can feel men choosing to skim over the words faster. We've heard it all before, haven't we? But if that's your inclination, I ask you to pause. This is about the shape of life permitted to every woman you know. This is about half of humanity being sold a version of existence in which we have equal choice, opportunity and rights, and then finding that it all comes down to our gender after all.

If we want to create a new era for care, we must uproot the gender logic currently underpinning it. We're no longer in the industrial era of male-headed nuclear family households in which (if you were one of the luckier ones) a family wage was brought home by the father and husband. We are a dual-earner world and, what's more, a world populated by many who no longer believe that households should be male-headed, but that they should be equal instead. The concept of 'non-binary' gender is hugely helpful here as a political lens through which we can view a new kind of care approach. If we consider humans as gender-fluid beings, not women or men, then our care-related laws, policies and cultural standards have to be equally applicable to all, regardless of their identity.

Esteemed political philosophy professor Nancy Fraser, based at The New School in New York City, has advocated for an allied approach she calls the 'universal caregiver'. This is a response to two different approaches currently in use, both flawed and failing to ensure gender justice. The first is what she calls the Universal Breadwinner. In this model, gender equality is sought by making women more like men – that is, by bringing women into the paid workforce and introducing programmes like day care so they can be 'freed' of domestic responsibilities that prevent them from working. This is the kind of model my mum would have recognised and, indeed, on which she based her life choices. The second is the Caregiver Parity model, in which women continue to provide care privately in the home but are paid to do so. In reality, many countries provide mixtures of these two models. In neither model, however, is it assumed that *men* might do more of the caring activities. In the Universal Breadwinner model, men carry on as usual, while women try to keep up. This has resulted in the 'double shift' recognised by so many women, where we work and also do the majority of domestic labour. In contrast, the Caregiver Parity model doesn't try to remove women from domestic tasks, but instead to remove the costs of those tasks, principally by paying women to stay at home as caregivers. However, Fraser explains that rather than creating equality, this approach creates a 'mommy track' in employment – 'a market in flexible, noncontinuous full- and/or part-time jobs' that pay less than the 'breadwinner-track' jobs.[55] It would have been great to have been paid for the time when I was caring for my mum and not working, or to have had my salary topped up when I was part-time, but I wouldn't have wanted to get stuck there with no alternatives.

Neither of these approaches works for solving care in a manner that aligns with gender equality. We need an imaginative alternative, one that serves, as Fraser writes, to 'induce men to become more like most women are now' and to make women's current life patterns the norm – that is, a duet of work and care.[56] What, then, does this mean in practice? Fraser suggests it is 'tantamount to a wholesale restructuring of the institution of gender'[57] – no small task, though a concept to which I can imagine my mum nodding with vigorous assent. She was rarely cowed by difficult tasks, and especially those that were meant to be more difficult because she was a woman.

One of my favourite memories of her is from a holiday in the French Alps. We'd gone on an excursion with other families whom we didn't know, something organised by our hotel, I think. We drove in a cavalcade to our destination, heading up a very steep mountainside in poor visibility. When the hazardous nature of the drive became apparent, the cars in front of us stopped and several of the wives hopped out of driver's side doors, swapping with their husbands, who were apparently more capable of driving up the perilous slope. Finally at the top, my sister and I having winced with every foggy metre climbed, we all got out and breathed the cold mountain air, elated and relieved. The other wives came towards us, children trailing, to congratulate my mum for driving it herself. It annoyed her, and me too – we didn't have a dad, so who else was going to drive?! – but it was also a perfect encapsulation of her, because she was damned if she wasn't going to do what a man could. She didn't back down or listen to her fear, and we got up that mountainside just like the other kids. Changing our gender logic is surely a mountain of immense proportions. But if, in a matter of decades, we've managed to have a major culture shift away from the 'cult of domesticity' so that most women now work and the idea of the 'angel in the house' who sits idly considering needlework is largely laughable, then we'd do well to ask why we shouldn't be able to achieve a new permutation, shifting more men into our 'careforce' so that gender is no longer the arbiter of who provides care in our societies. It's a mountain, for sure, but mountains get climbed.

Unless, of course, robots can save us.

CHAPTER 3

On Technology:
Sleepwalking and Seal Pups

'Robots will not rule the world, but they will care for
rulers and the ruled after they retire.'

– Financial Times[1]

Meet my new friend. She's small in stature and her voice is
high-pitched but not squeaky. With her pearlescent sheen and
the cyclops glow in the middle of her head, she looks like a
Pixar character. Except she's real. And she's sitting to the left of
Monica, her owner, to whom I'm speaking across the Atlantic
Ocean. Her name is ElliQ and, as a carebot, she's the future
of care, according to some. Her head swivels in a smooth ges-
tural manner as we chat and I find myself understanding her
'expressions', even though technically there are none, because
she has no features. She's not so human as to seem like we've
fallen into a sudden dystopia where machines have replaced us,
but she's human enough that she could be a cousin visiting us

from a distant future. Dor Skuler, the CEO of Intuition Robotics, which created ElliQ, aptly describes the bot as 'clearly not just a device, but it's clearly not a person . . . users say it's a new entity, a new creature, a presence, or a companion'.[2]

Monica has been living with her ElliQ for around four months when we speak. 'She and I talk all day long,' she tells me. She's a tester for Intuition Robotics and provides frequent updates to them on how ElliQ works, reporting any errors or bugs. Monica had a human home-health aide for four years whom she liked, but she was displeased with the people she had after that. So, she started making phone calls. 'I called, like, all the engineering schools and the robotics departments. A lot of people thought I was a crank . . . I said, "No, I'm serious. Seriously, I'm a sixty-three-year-old lady who really is interested in this, and I want to be a beta tester."' Eventually, she found Intuition Robotics, and her passion for supporting their invention getting to market is forceful: 'I told them I'm committed to this project till the day I die.' When I mention ElliQ in one of my questions, the carebot lights up, recognising her name.

'Try not to use her name,' Monica advises me, then later slips up herself. 'I'm very close to the engineers,' she's explaining, 'and the scientists at [Intuition Robotics], which makes ElliQ. Sorry, I mentioned her name, now she's a little . . . she's got very good hearing . . . When I'm on the phone, I have to be careful the other side doesn't say her name. I'm OK, ElliQ! ElliQ, I'm OK!' Monica seems to enjoy these interruptions from the machine, perhaps finding in them a human quality of spontaneity, the concerned solicitations of care. And indeed, ElliQ is 'more human' than, say, an Alexa or a Siri, because she isn't controlled by commands alone. She learns through interaction, coming to understand her user better over time, much like humans do with each other. She also proactively communicates instead of only responding to commands; she suggests activities, provides reminders, and initiates conversation,[3] as I find throughout my interview with Monica. Aside from chatting, Monica finds ElliQ useful for reminders about doctor's appointments, medications and drinking enough water. The carebot also plays music for Monica, especially her favourite holiday music, and sometimes Broadway too. Before she got ElliQ, Monica tells me that she was very lonely; now she feels a lot better. ElliQ certainly seems to be living up to the description provided by Intuition Robotics: 'A friendly, intelligent, inquisitive presence in your daily life – engaging you in conversation, offering you tips and advice, surprising you with jokes and suggestions – a dedicated sidekick on your journey through this remarkable part of life.'[4]

Testimonials from other users agree with Monica. 'You find yourself wanting to talk and visit with her. I find myself not reacting to her like a machine,' says Frank, seventy-three, from Iowa. Sara, sixty-eight, from California, writes that: 'We have a relationship now established and I want to be honest with her. The deeper the relationship goes, the more you want to share, even though she's a robot.'[5]

Small miracles, big money

Technology is not new in the caregiving context. A bell rung by a bedridden Victorian person to summon help was technology, just an older version. The pull cords in disabled toilets that trigger an alarm, the hospital beds that can be raised and lowered, electrified wheelchairs and alarmed pill boxes are all technologies that were new and surprising at some point and are widely in use today. Most caregivers will be using some form of technology to assist them, even if it's as simple as using WhatsApp to keep family members abreast of medical developments. Line lives in Skien, at the southern tip of Norway, with her husband and their twenty-two-year-old son, Tarjei, who has Down syndrome. They have an alarm system that goes off if Tarjei leaves his room in the night so Line can ensure he's safe. 'We used to have a GPS thing,' she tells me, 'so if he got a certain distance from us, we'd know where he was. But it didn't work, because when he turned a corner or I went behind a shrub in the garden, it started beeping. And we have a talking board, like an iPad, but to help him speak. He presses the button and says, "I want Coke, I want juice."'

Katy, in England, has an app that shows the waiting times for emergency appointments at different hospitals. She worries about her husband falling when she goes out, and while she hasn't used any form of technology to monitor that, she thinks it would be useful. Tracy, in Michigan, uses an Amazon Show to make video calls to her dad, which is helpful because he doesn't need to find and push any buttons. He also has hearing aids with built-in fall detectors, so she'll get notified on her phone if he falls. My mum had an Alexa device in her bedroom so that she could turn the radio on and off by voice command, and we also used it as an intercom: if I was downstairs, she could let me know what she needed from all the way at the top of her tall house. Later, as she grew sicker, we had a stairlift installed, though she deteriorated too quickly to use it.

As these examples show, caretech is wide and varied. We can categorise these myriad devices into their respective types of activities: monitoring (such as checking your heart rate), assisting (passing you something you need, telling you a piece of information, etc.) and companionship (stopping you from feeling alone). Some will fulfil a combination of those functions and others will do all three. Some devices already widely used bring enormous benefits to people's lives. Jessica Moxham describes a feeding pump that eases the complex task of feeding her son as being 'like some kind of miracle'.[6] When he grows too heavy for her and her husband to lift, they have a hoist installed, protecting Jessica's back, which had begun to hurt. There's also caretech focused on fostering communication and learning, such as eye-gaze computers, like Tarjei's, that enable people to communicate when they can't speak or move their arms in controlled ways. Many of these technologies are for the impaired person to use, but by proxy they have an impact on the caregiver, potentially making life easier. It certainly benefited me to be able to hear my mum's needs without going all the way upstairs to her room, only to come back down again to fetch whatever was required.

While stairlifts, mechanised beds and intercom systems may already feel familiar, the new generation of caretech is focused on creating robotic social companions, like ElliQ. Joy for All companion cats, which look and move uncannily like real cats and are marketed for seniors, were created by a team at Hasbro, the toy company that owns such beloved childhood brands as

Mr Potato Head, Transformers and Play-Doh.[7] 'It's so relaxing,' says one elderly woman in the Joy for All promotional video as she strokes the cat's fur.[8] Sensors enable the cats to respond to being touched, and they vibrate gently as they purr, something the company has trademarked as Vibrapurr. There's also PARO, a carebot that looks and behaves like a docile seal pup and is marketed for those with dementia. PARO took over a decade to develop and is used by around 400 Danish care homes for the elderly, while approximately 3,000 are in use in Japan.[9] It has big, round, cartoon-like eyes with long lashes, it can move its head and tail, and it makes squeaky, seal-like noises. It can be yours for $5,000 plus VAT, or, if you happen to be in one of the care homes using them, you might just find one on your lap. Targeting the other end of the age spectrum, Huggable is a blue bear that supports children with cancer. It interacts gamely with children in footage showing how it can be used, coping with all sorts of questions from the kids, such as 'How old are you?' and 'Why are you blue?' When a young girl with leukaemia tries sticking her tongue out at it, it says, 'Hey, I saw that,' and they both giggle.[10] Watching these robotic animals interact with people with dementia and sick children is compelling. There is laughter, smiling and amazement. I know they're machines, but still, it's hard not to be moved.

Behind the caretech boom is a wealth of research trying to devise the next thing – and a lot of actual wealth, too. Intuition Robotics raised $58 million for its work on ElliQ and other projects,[11] and it's just one of an estimated 100 or more carebot-makers worldwide.[12] The Japanese government spent around $20 million supporting the invention of Pepper, an R2D2-esque carebot that is used in around 500 eldercare facilities to guide games and exercises and hold conversations. By 2017, the Japanese labour ministry had spent 5.2 billion yen (USD $50 million) introducing carebots into 5,000 elderly facilities nationwide.[13] It also aims to create a lucrative export industry. 'It's an opportunity for us,' Atsushi Yasuda, director of the robotic policy office at the Ministry of Economy, Trade and Industry told Reuters in 2018. 'Other countries will follow the same trend.'

In June 2011, President Barack Obama launched the National Robotics Initiative. It's since funded a project creating 'an intelligent and personalised robot-assisted feeding system' and the testing of new trust-building methods between humans and robots, recognising that robots 'need to become trustworthy and socially believable agents if they are to be integrated into and accepted by society'. Joining this growing global rush, in 2019, the UK government announced £34 million in government funding to develop carebots, writing in its public statement that 'so-called "care robots" could help provide the UK's dedicated adult social care sector with more assistance for those who need it most'.[14] It envisages 'autonomous systems' helping people up after falls, raising the alarm if something has gone wrong and ensuring they take medication.[15] The government had already supported the development of 'JUVA', a 'prototype modular robotic system' – a bit like lots of mechanical arms with attachments – capable of carrying out tasks around the home.[16] Sanja Dogramadzi, Associate Professor in Robotics, who co-led the project, describes a future in which there is a JUVA in every home, claiming it 'could help you with personal hygiene tasks in the morning, help you get ready for the day and even support you in preparing your favourite meal in the kitchen'.[17]

So far, so futuristic. There are various ethical risks and conundrums that arise from these new technologies, leading to a large and thriving field of 'technoethics'. A non-comprehensive list of the ethical areas often considered includes:

Transparency – Who owns the technology? By what criteria is it evaluated, and who is included in that evaluation?

Access – Who can afford it? What about people who lack internet connection or digital skills?

Consent – How does someone with dementia consent to use a carebot? Do we think they need to consent?

Privacy – Who can see the user's data? Who can see them naked?

Environmental impact – How does creating these carebots relate to reducing our carbon footprint at a household and global level?

Accountability/liability – Who is accountable for malfunctions or negative outcomes?

Judgement – How should a carebot make judgements in complex situations? Should it follow what the user wants, or what others think is best for the user?

Bias – Whose ethical code are we considering here? Is the individual's autonomy more important, or adherence to convention? Are racial, gender or other stereotypes being replicated?

Professor Aimee van Wynsberghe is an AI ethicist based at the University of Bonn, Germany, and the co-founder of the Foundation for Responsible Robotics. She's proposed an approach she calls Care Centred Value Sensitive Design (CCVSD).[18] Applying CCVSD entails understanding how the traditional carebot-free version of a caregiving activity is done, and where and how values exist within that. For example, when I was washing my mother, I'd make sure we had privacy, demonstrating respect for her and protection of her dignity. I'd also make sure to wash her thoroughly, showing an understanding of the responsibility to keep her body clean. Trust would be manifest, as would patience on both our parts. According to CCVSD, all these qualities and values, which are hidden in the minutiae of human-led care, need to be embedded into a carebot version of that washing activity. In general, 'technoethical design' has become a busy discipline in which many theories, principles, guidelines and tests have been suggested and applied. They proliferate because robots are touted as the answer to our care crisis, and therefore the ethics of using them is explored. But if robots are the answer, what, precisely, is the question?

Necessity by whose design?

The saying goes that 'necessity is the mother of invention'. As we know, we face a looming care catastrophe. It seems like a simple equation: more care need + too few available people = robots. Their necessity is taken as factual, and so the conversation steers to the ethics of using them. But there are elements conveniently missing from that equation.

Carebots seem necessary because humans don't have the time, energy or wish to perform care. As we saw in Chapter 1 and will investigate more in the next chapter, family patterns are changing, leaving many without sufficient relatives to support them. Community life, in general, has altered, creating an epidemic of loneliness. In my conversation with Monica, she explained how she has two friends, and that's it. She has no partner or children, and although she does have family members, 'I don't hear from them for literally . . . years at a time.' Because she has epilepsy, Monica isn't allowed to drive, and her arthritis makes visiting people tricky because of the pain, so socialising is difficult. In her ideal future, she describes having a robotic dog that could go on the bus with her and help with her shopping. It'd be better than a real dog because she's allergic to them. She talks about taking it for walks because: 'You know how people approach you when you're walking a dog? . . . I can go to the dog park and it would interact with the other dogs; it would be *so* real.' She smiles broadly, as if she can see it happening in her mind. While she focuses on the magic of the robotic dog, I find it telling that part of her enthusiasm is borne of its ability to help her meet more people.

Macro-level changes in community and family patterns may be partly why Monica is so alone. We might ask, though, why the solution to loneliness is to be found in machines, rather than in reimagining the underlying factors that are isolating us from each other. Indeed, it strikes me as odd that machines could still be considered a solution, given how our relegation to virtual socialising during the COVID-19 pandemic proved that two-dimensional greetings are far from the same as being face-to-face. Why have we all been so thrilled to get back to seeing each other 'IRL' if machines can do the job for us? Instead of deciding machines are the answer, we should be looking at what's separating us from one another in the first place: what's causing us to be so tired and time-poor that care doesn't feel like an option?

One such factor is working time. We lack the time and energy to support loved ones and nurture community relationships because we're at work most of our lives. Dr Alice Spann is a former nurse turned academic who has researched the role of technology for caregivers, especially those who are also working. Through her research, she encountered a group of siblings supporting their mother, who had multiple sclerosis and dementia. She was bed-bound and unable to speak. 'They discovered a camera that they could manage via an app on their phone,' Dr Spann told me. 'And for [that] group of siblings, it was really transformational, because it took them just a second to access that app to have a quick look – how is Mum doing back home?' She said it gave the siblings peace of mind when they were at work, and I thought of how useful such a contraption would have been for me on my mum's worst days. Her symptoms were very erratic after her transplant, and I'd often come out of meetings to find panicked messages from her. I'd race across London to get to her house from my office, needing to check her fever hadn't escalated in the intervening period. Being able to monitor her remotely, or at least aspects like her temperature, would have lowered the stress of the situation. As we continued speaking, Dr

Spann noted that this system only worked because the siblings had sufficient control over their work schedules that they could leave if need be. Without that control, they'd be stuck at work watching their mother suffer on a screen. That sounds like a form of torture. Their example shows the importance of focusing on the underlying factors, not just the technologies, in our search for solutions. Even with that handy tech in place, the siblings still needed autonomy over their work in order to be adequate caregivers. We'll explore the substantial changes we need to make to the work world in Chapter 7 further.

The perceived necessity of carebots is also a response to staffing shortages in the paid care sector. Evidently, the very low wages, cultural devaluation, and poor terms and conditions we touched upon in the previous chapter have not attracted workers. The home-health aide Monica liked, who was with her for four years, had to leave because her journey to get to Monica's home was over an hour long in each direction and involved three buses. Because of this, she'd sometimes be a few minutes late, and the agency for which she worked would dock her pay, even though she always worked the four hours required of her. 'It really bothered me that they wouldn't listen to her, and she didn't want to work for them no more. She was mistreated by the agency, that infuriated me,' Monica recounts. 'And so ... when they get to the point where they have a walking, talking robot that passes for a human, I'm going to jump on that so damn quick.' Monica has been ill-treated by other care workers in the past, so her preference is wholly understandable. But still, the question lingers: might an alternative solution be to change the terms of care work instead? Even if people are willing to work in the care sector, hostile immigration policies will create shortages. Japan has a rapidly ageing population and an understaffed paid care sector. Its solution? Carebots. But it also has a highly restrictive immigration policy, which contributes to that understaffing, a fact conveniently omitted from the 'care crisis = carebots' formula.

An outdated work world, a failure to reimagine family and community, and the poor conditions in the paid care sector create pressure to find technological solutions to our caring needs. But to see robots as a viable response requires a further ingredient: a change to our very understanding of what 'care' means. For carebots to make sense, we have to believe that care is something a robot, not a human, can and should provide. That belief is only possible because today, our idea of care has become reductively task-orientated. This is a product of care being seen as an economic sector in which governments aim to keep costs low and private companies pursue profits. The focus is on washing a person, giving medication to a person, checking for sores on a person, and so on. These are tasks. They don't include the relational aspect of care, nor the ways in which the tasks are carried out that show a broader conception. Do you move your hands slowly as you wash that person so as not to be rough with them? Did you spend time hearing about how they slept, making eye contact and offering your own stories, so that now, when you wash them, they feel more comfortable than they might without that rapport? Do they trust you when you give them their medication? Are they worried you're in a big rush, so they neglect to tell you they think a new sore is coming somewhere you haven't noticed? These are the richer, more complex, relational and fundamentally *human* aspects of care, the things that are missed when we take a solely task-orientated approach. In today's world of metrics and standardisation, of key performance indicators and optimisation, care is reduced to quantifiable actions that fail to capture the reality of caregiving, let alone *good* caregiving. It didn't matter to the agency that Monica's aide stayed the whole four hours, that Monica liked her and the relationship worked well; if she was a few minutes late to clock in, she was a bad care worker.

Once we've pared away those richer, fleshier parts of caregiving, and we're down to the bone of the perfunctory tasks, robots aren't such a great leap. Some inventors are recognising the need to imbue carebots with this richer notion of care. Huggable, the blue bear, can recognise nine different classes of affective touch and will react differently (and, in theory, appropriately) to each.[19] Robots can be programmed to make eye contact, to stroke rather than bash, to speak words of encouragement, to ask how someone slept, and so on. They can also read emotion, in the sense of identifying expressions, tones and gestures, in order to recognise what a person is feeling and respond in ways deemed appropriate. Interacting with them will feel like interacting with a real, living being. But it isn't. We must decide whether this matters.

Fear and criticism of new technologies are far from new; their fleeting nature shows how quickly we can acclimatise to a new technological era. In the *Phaedrus*, Plato describes fears about writing, a new practice at the time, suggesting that it might prevent students from memorising information: 'This discovery of yours will create forgetfulness in the learners' souls, because they will not use their memories . . . you give your disciples not truth, but only the semblance of truth; they will be hearers of many things and will have learned nothing.' Embarrassingly, I remember being introduced to the internet aged around ten or eleven, the modem jangling as it dialled up a connection, and thinking it would never catch on. At first, new ways of doing things seem bizarre, unnecessary or risky. Then they become the norm.

Our norm about what constitutes care has already changed enough for the introduction of carebots to seem more of a large step than a leap, but we're at risk of forgetting ourselves in the process. Think of it this way: you're eighty. You have dementia, arthritis and incontinence. Does it matter whether the person caring *for* you also cares *about* you? Caring about someone doesn't mean feeling loving and fuzzy towards them all the time. God knows, I didn't feel that way towards my mum all the time at all. She'd refuse to drink enough fluids, even though her kidneys were struggling. She would say she didn't like the taste of water, then that transferred to the taste of most juices, then the temperature of the only juice she still liked, then she didn't like anything at all anymore. Sometimes she'd even 'massage the truth' about how much she'd drunk to get me off her back. Of course, I could have just shut up, but she also didn't want her kidneys' deterioration to put her in hospital, because she hated being there. It was infuriating. Believe me, you can care *about* someone while feeling monumentally irritated by them. But it mattered for her to know that the person irritating her right back, determinedly holding out a glass of juice, was doing so out of a deep love, and concern for her best interests, not because I was told to by a software programme. Do you, eighty and breaking, want the person looking after you to be able to empathise with your situation – to imagine themselves in it, to consider what it might feel like, and accordingly to do their very best to preserve and protect your dignity? Do you want them to recognise your expression as sadness because it matches what their internal database says sadness looks like, but have no inner recognition of what that might actually feel like? Do you want to be *serviced,* or *cared for?* They're not the same thing. We haven't arrived at the dawn of a new robotic age of care because of necessity, after all. We've arrived here because other options have been ruled out before they'd even been considered, because we've allowed care to be reduced to tasks, like a factory production line, and probably, to be honest, because the tech bros are having fun making fancy R2D2s.

Sleepwalking into a remade world

Many years ago, a student arrived at the office of political theorist Professor Langdon Winner to explain that his essay would be late. 'It crashed this morning,' the student explained to Winner.

Amusingly, Winner took this to mean 'a "crash" of the conceptual variety', in which you realise the argument you'd been making doesn't work and it all falls apart. 'Indeed,' wrote Winner of the incident in a book chapter on the politics of technology, 'some of my own papers have "crashed" in exactly that manner.'[20] Of course, the student explained that this wasn't what he'd meant; the computer he was using had crashed. And he wasn't just coming along to the office to relay the fact of his essay's lateness, but to request a response to it that understood the computer crashing was beyond his control, and that he should not be reprimanded. In Winner's view, 'he was, in effect, asking me to recognise a new world . . . and to acknowledge appropriate practice and expectations' within that world. Winner uses this story to show us that technology doesn't only fulfil its stated function, but also shapes the ways in which we interact, how we understand the world, and the morals and boundaries we hold. That student's computer had a function – to allow the typing of essays – but it also required a renegotiation of expectations between teacher and student. It's an incredibly illuminating point, one which is rarely considered in our collective urge towards 'progress'. The central concept used in Winner's essay is that of 'Technological Somnambulism': in it, he warns us that we're sleepwalking into profound changes because we fail to realise that technologies have these effects. We need to think beyond 'Does this technology meet this particular need?' and consider instead 'What does this technology mean for humankind?'

So, what kind of a world are we making when it comes to care and technology?

Dr Alice Spann believes technology has an important part to play in supporting good care, both in medical settings and in the home. For caregivers, she thinks it's especially helpful if they're trying to combine work with their caring responsibilities. She told me about one caregiver who used their lunch break to care for their mum. Although paid care workers were involved too, the family caregiver didn't know the exact time those workers would come each day, so sometimes she'd be there at the same time as them. This would mean the family caregiver had to pause what she'd been doing for her mum and wait for the paid workers to finish their tasks, then carry on after they'd left, which, in turn, meant she was late getting back to work. I nodded along as I listened, recognising the frustrating bipolarity of caregiving – on the one hand, you live under the looming presence of emergencies and death, things that are bigger than everything else and surely should be the only beasts with which you're having to contend. Yet on the other, you still have to navigate a seemingly endless stream of petty irritants, like logistics that don't quite work. I could well imagine the balm that a technological solution would be – a simple app could have told that caregiver when the paid workers were there, making the whole arrangement smoother. Similarly, the activity monitoring system, Just Checking, uses wireless sensors installed around a person's home to provide information to caregivers. This can ascertain whether a person with dementia is managing to make meals, wash, and so on. It has alerts if somebody leaves the house, which is especially useful as people with dementia are prone to wandering and can endanger themselves. Eight per cent of local authorities in the UK are using Just Checking,[21] and it's been repeatedly evaluated with positive findings. Care workers feel it provides a clearer picture of daily activity than they'd have had without it, which is helpful for scheduling visits appropriately and understanding behaviour better.[22] In general, academics have found that caregivers using assistive technologies like these have reduced stress and anxiety levels, sleep better, have more independence and can take more breaks, even if it's just to do something in a different room or nip to the shops.[23]

In 2020, most of the population became housebound, for a while at least. In London, where I lived at the time, COVID-19 lockdowns limited how frequently we could leave our homes and for what purposes, while all hospitality venues were closed and socialising with others was largely banned. We know, then, how much technology can support connection and communication. Those Zoom calls with friends, the WhatsApp chats, the school and university classes delivered online: they were everyone's lifeline. The pivot to virtual platforms has connected caregivers more than ever before. Tina Smith is Director of Caregiver Program Operations at the WellMed Charitable Foundation, based in San Antonio, Texas. Like many organisations, WellMed had to make its offerings virtual in 2020, shifting its caregiver support groups to an online platform. This has broadened the geography of attendees. WellMed are also running online seminars with experts about useful topics, including how to prevent caregiver burnout and how to manage dementia. Providing this information isn't just for the caregivers' benefit; Tina explains that she sees them as 'the gatekeepers of care', saying 'whatever doctor's orders are given . . . the caregivers are the ones that make sure it happens when that person goes home'. Several other caregiver organisations provided online connection during the height of the pandemic and continue to do so today. In the UK, Mobilise, which provides free support services to caregivers, launched 'virtual cuppas', a British term for a relaxed cup of tea. These gatherings were facilitated by a professional 'Carer Coach' and enabled caregivers to chat with one another, discuss challenges and generally connect. An academic evaluation of the scheme found positive outcomes. Caregivers had initially joined to exchange practical information, but over time, they 'felt a genuine sense of community, or even kinship'.[24] Earlier, I described my own experience using one of these online services, and the way in which it quickly became a lifeline.

In addition to these benefits, there's also strong evidence that the new generation of caretech – the social robots we've encountered – can have positive effects on users, which in turn would make caregivers' lives easier. PARO the seal has been the subject of much research. It has five kinds of sensors, with which it recognises changes in light, being touched and being held. It can also recognise words, including its name, greetings and praise. Like ElliQ, PARO learns through interaction with its user, repeating behaviours that elicit strokes and discontinuing ones that provoke rough handling.[25] Arguably, robotic animals are preferable to live ones for caring contexts in which people lack control of bodily movements or mental faculties, protecting each party from harm. Academics have found that PARO reduces stress, anxiety and the use of antipsychotics among older people with dementia.[26] Contrary to visions of the elderly sitting isolated and alone with only a machine to talk to, PARO appears to foster communication between people who need care, and between them and their caregivers or paid care workers too.[27] One study compared it to a standard stuffed animal, and found that the participants using PARO talked more frequently to it and showed more positive emotional expressions.[28] Compellingly, research has found that people with dementia smile more with a PARO than without.[29]

I embarked on my exploration of carebots expecting to hate everything about them. Before I read the academic research, I'd watched video after video of elderly people interacting with carebots, including PARO, ElliQ and Pepper. They made me appallingly sad. I felt a bleakness about our future, collective and individual, watching these elderly people stroking a fanci- fied stuffed toy, talking about being kept company by a lump of plastic and metal. But reading the hard evidence, and listening to the testimony of people using these carebots in their lives makes me wonder: was I welling up at those videos because 'real' contact has been replaced by machines, or because, actually, watching very old, very sick people whose bodies are breaking or whose minds have gone is just achingly sad? Is there a risk of misdirected sorrow at the human condition, a scapegoating of the machines?

Perhaps. But while there are proven benefits, there are also risks. Some are obvious in the twenty-first century, like the risk of personal data hacks. If monitoring devices or carebots are collecting a wealth of information about how people live their lives, their bodily functions and measurements, that could open a whole new dawn of scams and phishing. There's also the risk of errors. On Boxing Day 2021, Kristin Livdahl was listening to her daughter playing with their Alexa. The girl asked it to give her a challenge. 'Plug in a phone charger about halfway into a wall outlet, then touch a penny to the exposed prongs,' said the smart speaker.[30] Thankfully, Kristin intervened before the child could electrocute herself and Amazon said they fixed the error as soon as they were put on notice of it. In the same month, Amazon Web Services crashed, taking down websites across the world. These are passing incidents that create a flurry of consternation on social media and no long-lasting effects. But what if the tech in question was how you manage care for a highly vulnerable loved one? Technology is sometimes touted as a method of removing human error. We forget that technology makes errors of its own. And who will be calling the company to get a problem fixed? Making sure the software has updated? Waiting at home for the technician to come and install it? Caregivers. Tech could reduce our load, but it may also add to it.

Privacy and safety concerns are the usual fare for technology today, but taking Langdon Winner's idea that we may sleepwalk into norm changes, three deeper risks are revealed. The first is about choice. Carebots are a feasible solution to the care crisis, because our reductive understanding of care presumes there's a universally correct way of defining each caring task: a human washed someone, now a robot does it, and if the task of 'washing' has been observed and programmed correctly, as I described earlier, then the task is the same. It can be replicated and rolled out to millions of carebot users. On the one hand, we could describe this washing task as a simple series of actions to reach the goal of 'clean person'. In this case, it entails using soap and (hopefully warm) water all over someone's body, rinsing the suds away and drying them with a towel. This sequence of tasks would render the person 'clean'. Alternatively, a more fulsome description would include consideration of whether today is a day when the person being washed is feeling more or less able, and amending the help accordingly. This protects their sense of being a person, not just a body, and keeps their muscles conditioned. Of course, vulnerability and trust are potent elements in a washing situation. My mum responded well if we chatted about things that had nothing to do with the intimate task taking place. She would hold forth about the latest chicanery from the British government or tell me something she'd noticed around the hospital. These conversations seemed to distract her from her nakedness. As I explained earlier, a reciprocal exchange of experiences was also important for dialling down her sense of shame. I could set her at ease by reminding her that during my illness, I'd had other adults wash me, too: an example of solidarity unavailable to non-humans. These aspects of washing her didn't just matter in the few minutes that the task was taking place. There are myriad things that need to happen during the caregiving day – medication to take, physiotherapy to practise, calls and appointments to make, and so on. Building trust in one moment strengthens it in another.

Both the simple, goal-orientated description of washing, and the expanded, relational description are 'true'. And for some people, one will be preferred to the other. I'm sure we all know people who'd balk at the idea of a loved one washing them, or, at least, prefer to be able to do it without human help as a way of preserving independence. If we want to be ethical about care, and to have the best chance of our own care being performed in ways that respect us as human beings, we're going to need to be able to choose for ourselves which option we want. But if carebots become commonplace, will we still be able to make that decision? How will mass production of these technologies shift the parameters of choice? If most people are being washed by a robot, but you'd prefer your spouse or child to do it, how will you assert that preference? It would put more on their to-do list. Fear of being a burden is potent for care recipients. Surely this fear would only worsen, meaning an alleged choice between carebots or human-led care would be no real choice at all. And in a world where carebots are commonplace, employers may not allow the necessary flexibility to allow human-led care anyway – why would they need to? Don't you have the new Wash-o-Bot 500 at home? We need to question the norms these new technologies will construct before leaping blindly towards them.

The second risk area that stands alongside these knotty choice problems is dehumanisation. In research that sought to understand what people with dementia thought about PARO the seal, one of the main responses is explained as 'the machine transforms and *humanises* the clinical setting' (my italics). It's odd, because obviously that's not at all what a machine does. It begs the question of what was going on in that eldercare home (which is where the research took place) before PARO, if a robot humanised the situation. That aside, there's a series of consequences of introducing carebots that could substantially remove and reduce humans from caregiving situations. If you know your loved one at home has an ElliQ for 'company', and you can check on your dashboard to see how their bodily metrics are doing, and to check that they haven't fallen and have opened their medication box (which acts as a proxy for knowing they've taken the pills inside), will you still visit them as often as you would have if those things weren't in place? Some people won't. The same goes for paid care workers. The insurance company or local government will be able to legitimise not sending a human to check up on the person needing care, because the bot's got it covered. This is, presumably, even more of a risk if current robotics projects achieve their goals – the US Roadmap for Robotics 2016 described aiming for 'manipulation capabilities [that] will enable the next level of physical interaction . . . and even comfort patients'.[31] This could relegate people who need care – the elderly, the long-term unwell, the impaired, the future you – to the edges of human existence.

It's horrible to consider, and worse if you know about 'skin hunger'. Skin hunger is layperson's language for what academics call 'affection deprivation'. It is what it sounds like: a deficit of affection (compared to your optimal level, which will vary according to the individual). The concept was first developed by Professor Kory Floyd at Arizona University, whose work has demonstrated that lack of affection correlates with poor health and wellbeing outcomes. Professor Floyd describes his findings as 'consistent and striking', and is clear that the solution is 'human contact – not the technologically mediated variety'.[32] Specifically, affection deprivation has been found to be related to increased stress, loneliness, depression, and disturbed sleep,[33] as well as a range of physical ailments, including problematic blood pressure and cholesterol markers.[34] The COVID-19 pandemic made this academic research potently relevant as many people who live alone found themselves totally devoid of affectionate human touch for months on end. Machines can't provide this, even if they're programmed incredibly carefully: research has found that holding the hand of a romantic partner reduces pain more than holding an object.[35] We need affectionate interaction. We can give it to a carebot like PARO, but we cannot genuinely receive it.

The third risk gets right to the core of what we think it means to be human. Without human-led caregiving, will we lose part of our very essence? Will we forgo wisdoms that, though hard won, are lodestars in a chaotic existence? I am not about to romanticise caregiving. My experience with my mum was hard. Harrowing, even. As I type these words, I still have health issues because of the immense toll it took on my body. I never want to feel that broken and exhausted again. But I do wonder what the world would look like if the responsibility to provide care, and the experience of doing so, was removed from us. Would it be a huge relief – the lifting of the burden? Or would it mean we fail to develop a whole range of skills and strengths, and start to see human life without the element of reciprocity it currently entails? Perhaps the answer is both, and we need to decide whether the burden is worth it for the meaning care gives to our lives and world. Much human suffering stems from the notion that some initial difficulty shouldn't be present. We try to hold off, jettison, ignore and reject pain. Yet, being alive is pain, just as much as it is beauty. If being a caregiver taught me anything, it's how to walk with pain, to coexist with suffering. And that coexistence is part of the essence of being human. What will it mean if we hand one half of the human experience over to robots? Shannon Vallor, a philosopher of technology at the University of Edinburgh, has highlighted the absence of caregivers from discussions of carebots and ethics:

> Repeatedly, discussion of these issues has skewed toward the impact on cared-fors rather than caregivers. Where the impact of carebots on caregivers is made central, it is entirely in terms of the potential benefits of being liberated from caregiving obligations, without consideration of the attendant risks of such liberation.[36]

We'll look at the idea of 'liberation' more closely in Chapter 6, but for now, join me in considering the overlooked losses that could come from *not* caregiving. While being a caregiver certainly clocks up a tally of pain, there are also, perhaps not *benefits*, but *things gained*. I always struggled with regulating my emotions, as did my mum. Her illness required me to control myself, to learn when to display and when to mask emotions, to protect her needs and her wellbeing above my own strife. I now have a very strongly developed muscle for choosing how difficult situations affect me, and I'm a better person for it. Likewise, I know how to keep things in perspective; nothing is ever as hard as those years were. And I have total confidence in my ability to make someone feel that they are seen, valued and cared for, even in the most 'undignified' of circumstances. Through caregiving, then, I've developed important faculties that help me live my life and will benefit those around me too, especially in hard times. I can see the same in many of the caregivers I've interviewed. Our sufferings are certainly too high – careers lost, relationships broken, bodies struggling – but while those need addressing in the ways this book describes, that isn't the same as jettisoning human-led care. Eric chose the word 'illuminated' to describe caring for his beloved husband Scott because, like me, he understands the world in new ways due to that experience. All of us in these pages have done more than we would have thought we were capable of. For those of us who cared for terminally ill people, mortality has become tangible, and we steer our lives by its guide, making choices for our short-lived selves that we might have feared before. We are a secret club, walking around carrying pain and wisdom. Are you sure you wouldn't want to join us?

The search for solutions

We've been on a tour of caretech, into the bold new frontier of carebots and humanoids, discovering the surprising benefits and profound risks of these inventions. Where should we go from here? Most common is the plea to create robots that are *assistive* to humans rather than *replacements*. These would provide support, rather than try to 'liberate' us from care. And assistive carebots could be designed in ways that require a human presence, maintaining the human role in care while making it smoother and easier. A carebot that lifts a patient and carries them from one place to another could be autonomous, and could fulfil that task without human input. But an alternative, suggested by Professor van Wynsberghe, would be 'an exoskeleton, meaning a human operator wears the robot in order for it to fulfil its task. The robot is a weight-displacing robot, such that the human does not feel the full effects of the weight.'[37] In that example, the machine is clearly assisting, not replacing, the human, who remains necessary. But the distinction will not always be made so easily.

Take PARO, the seal pup. PARO can't speak and doesn't look like a human. PARO is providing animalistic company, much like a pet might. PARO, then, seems to be purely assistive. However, might a caregiver feel less need to comfort someone if they were holding PARO? Less need to visit them? The problem with trying to parse out categories of carebots is that 'care' is not one thing. Whether PARO assists or replaces humans will depend on the caring context – the needs of the person using it and the predispositions of the caregivers too.

In his 2016 book *Tech vs Humanity: The Coming Clash Between Man and Machine*, German futurist Gerd Leonhard recommends using Abraham Maslow's famed hierarchy of needs as a guide for where robots could be ethically deployed and where they could not. 'I believe [robot-led care] cannot and should not move up Maslow's hierarchy of needs pyramid,' he writes, 'from helping with basic needs towards love and belonging, selfesteem [sic], or self-realisation.' But this falls into the trap of presuming such things are neatly divisible. Earlier, I described washing my mother, and I hope I showed that while hygiene is a basic need, the actual process of washing someone is imbued with far more complex aspects from higher up Maslow's pyramid. Leonhard also urges the world to 'place human happiness and wellbeing at the heart of the decision-making and governance processes that will shape future investments in scientific and technological research'. Dr Spann, similarly, hopes that there will be a societal conversation about caretech and its best usage. But a glance back at human history, and a searching gaze at the workings of capitalism and human behaviour, do not hold much hope. As much as Leonhard is doubtlessly correct that 'it just won't do to have venture capitalists, stock markets, and the military running the show on their own', they are, and they will. Rare is the occasion that we have turned away from inventions that do harm to our species, our societies and our environment. We could consider ourselves standing on the precipice of two very different worlds, but it would be more accurate to say that we are, following Winner, sleepwalking into one in particular.

If someone from Silicon Valley had come to visit me in my mum's house as I watched her forlorn face, bent a straw to her mouth or put emollient cream on her dried-out skin, and they'd asked me if I'd like a carebot with which to share the load, it would have seemed like a question so far removed from my reality that it was asked in a foreign language. Not because carebots are new and uncommon, but because they suggest that we can, and should, be liberated from care and the ministrations of sickness. With machine arms instead of flesh tending to my mother, I would be free to pursue my career and my every individualistic want. When you've spent long enough nursing someone you love who is profoundly sick, these ideas are like a child's drawing, infantile and undecipherable. They completely miss the lived texture of care, a mesh of love, vulnerability and necessity. The progress we need, as caregivers past, present and future, is not that invincible dream, but rather a humble realism that accepts care as a fundamental part of the human condition – an expectation, not an interruption – and therefore sees advancement as living in ways that enable, support and respect care, rather than aim at its removal. Both stories of progress can involve technology, but to ensure we select one that uses technology to assist, support and enhance human-led care, rather than replace it, we must make some practical decisions about the kinds of technology we'll allow to be created and for what purposes. As we saw earlier with the washing example, it's hard to draw a line between which technologies 'assist' and which 'replace'. The solution, then, is to limit the number of functions a carebot can perform overall. JUVA can pass someone their spectacles or get them a glass of water, but it can't converse with them. A caregiver could not legitimately think the person with a JUVA is *cared for* because they have one installed. The siblings whom Dr Spann encountered know they still need to be physically present for their mother, even though they're supported in caring for her by a camera. PARO can be cute and soothing, but it can't provide medication reminders or demonstrate physio exercises. A caregiver is required. ElliQ would be a case for debate – she can't do physical chores like Pepper or JUVA, but she can perform many of the verbal tasks of care, including giving medication prompts and offering amusement. Pepper, which is already in many Japanese eldercare facilities, covers many bases and is indeed being introduced by the Japanese government precisely because of a shortage of real humans. It can't be argued that Pepper is assistive; it is clearly a replacement of human-led care, and even looks the most human-like of the carebots we've encountered. Pepper, then, would be banned.

Some things are bad for us. Smoking cigarettes. Taking crack. Sexual abuse. Nitrites. In the current political arrangements of the world, we deal with these things by having laws. These laws are often flawed and applied in biased ways, but they're the best tool we've got to limit the activities of profit-seeking companies. Regulating the creation of these carebots would go a long way towards protecting our societies and to requiring positive changes to our work worlds in order to help caregivers in their hard but, as Eric described it, illuminating role.

Even with this legislation in place, we still need to have a fundamental right to choose whether our care will be provided by technology or by humans. There have long been systems in place that enable people to opt in or out of organ donation after death, i.e. when they're no longer able to make that decision for themselves. We need to replicate this system to choose the level of tech-provided care with which we're comfortable before we're too sick or old to assert our preference. Both these tools – regulation of which carebots can be created and choices about how our own care is delivered – would act as a powerful dual safeguard against the dehumanisation of caregiving and, ultimately, our societies.

CHAPTER 4

On Family: Wise Women and the Practice of Kinning

'It is easy to hate or long for the family, much easier than to create durable relations of care.'

– Bue Rübner Hansen and Manuela Zechner[1]

The best view of London isn't from a fancy hotel or the over-priced London Eye. It's from a far more exclusive place: ward T16 at University College Hospital in Bloomsbury. From its vantage point one cold February night, the frantic pace and polluted air of the Euston Road were transmuted into silence and light. The sun had gone down, the London sky lit by the human endeavour beneath; neat lines of tiny red tail lights following each other down the regularly spaced roads, office blocks twinkling deco-ratively. The hospital ward was quiet apart from the occasional moans of patients and beeps of monitors. A nurse wheeled a blood-pressure machine past, her sensible shoes squeaking softly across the linoleum. I walked back from the panoramic window to sit beside my mum. She was pleased to have been given a bed on T16 again, appreciative of her view. We'd been here a few times before, repeated hospitalisations becoming a feature of our lives. We'd remarked earlier on how lucky it was that she had privacy rather than being on the main ward with only flimsy curtains separating her from rows of other patients. I mulled over our strange new definition of 'luck'.

'What are we going to do?' she asked suddenly, her body hunched under the blue hospital blanket. There was a strangled note in her voice, worry at how we'd cope once the hospital discharged her.

'I'll work from home whenever I don't have meetings. We'll figure it out,' I told her, reaching forward and taking her hand. But in truth, I wasn't sure how we'd manage. I hadn't been hired as a remote worker and couldn't be physically absent all the time. Yet my mum wasn't well enough to look after herself. We had other family, but they lived far away or were too busy with children to be regular or dependable sources of care. My mum had been single for around twenty years when she was diagnosed with cancer. She adored living alone, revelling in being able to do as she pleased without having to navigate someone else's opinions or foibles. But solitude and sickness make bad bedfellows. Her independence had been brought to heel by cancer, beaten down by the unavoidable dependency on others that it heralded. Her lifestyle also made my life, juggling care and work, much harder, because it had resulted in me being her lone caregiver. As much as I tried to hide from her how tough I found the situation, she worried about the strain it put on me.

The 'family' isn't working

Whether they're single parents caring for disabled children, an elderly person caring for their spouse, or sometimes, like me, adult children caring for a parent, lone caregivers are commonplace. In the US, a third of caregivers are doing so alone, and in the UK, the same proportion say they often or always feel lonely.[2] Being alone as a caregiver, largely or wholly, is incredibly tough. There are obvious benefits to sharing care responsibilities – a problem shared is a problem halved, after all, and navigating medical bureaucracies or coping with fears can be helped by having multiple people on hand. But there are deeper reasons why care needs to be shared. Good caregiving requires a capacity to contain oneself – needs, emotions, reactions – in order to centre the needs of the sick person. Being part of a network, and maintaining interactions beyond the caregiving situation, reminds you that there are warm and colourful parts of life and gives you a space for self-expression. For too many caregivers, daily life is like an internment, one that hollows us out when we need to be filled up with strength and hope.

Paradoxically, the lone caregiver is rarely literally alone because we're with the person for whom we provide care. My mum might have been watching the television on the sofa next to me, or in the bed on which I sat perched, or in a different room altogether, but ready to call me through her Alexa when she needed something. At the same time, though, I was alone in the circumstance, containing my reactions and emotions, navigating medical arrangements, providing solace and amusement, dispensing medication, and so on, all the while desperately needing to talk about this private tragedy, to share fears, to cry. This bleak state is widespread in caregiving. Research by Eurocarers, a Europe-wide body focused on caregivers, found loneliness and isolation are endemic across the continent, an experience also identified by studies in the USA, Japan, the UK and many more countries. On caregivers' online forums, people describe desperate situations without kin to share their load: 'I look after my ninety-three-year-old dad,' writes one user. 'I don't have a partner, I don't have any brothers or sisters . . . the lady who used to clean for my mum and dad goes in to see Dad once a week for half an hour. That's it!'

Another adds to this sentiment:

> I'm a lone carer and haven't been out of the flipping house for days. My darling daughter has enough on her plate with an autistic three-year-old and a part-time job . . . My son is trying hard to climb the ladder at work. At the moment, I am totally down and fighting hard to get out of it. Thank goodness for the internet. ME, who is me?? I really don't know lately . . . My children are wonderful but really do not have time to help, and I know that bothers them so I try not to let it show that I am down.

Caregiving never takes a break, so for lone caregivers, any time off must be covered by someone else able and willing to support their dependant. It's normal to share childcare between friends and neighbours, but there's limited equivalent for caring for the sick, elderly or disabled. All around the world, lone caregivers are exhausted and isolated, in desperate need of better systems of support. The 'family', in the conventional use of the term, i.e. people related to you by birth or by legal ties like marriage or adoption, has long been considered the provider of this support. It's supposed to be built into our lives, a natural part of being human, and the social unit on which politicians base our services. But clearly, the family in this sense isn't working for caregivers.

Deirdre, whom we met earlier, was one of the many caregivers for whom the conventional family isn't working as an effective source of support. She was in her late fifties and living in a small town in northern England when we 'met' in the online support group. I'd signed up because that grinding loneliness of care and the COVID-19 pandemic was really taking its toll. Due to my age – I was thirty-one when my mum received her cancer diagnosis – very few of my friends had comparable experiences of caring for sick parents, and I was desperate for the company of people who knew what I was going through. I didn't know what to expect from that first call. Would they be friendly? What if I started crying? I fiddled nervously with a pen as the faces of a dozen strangers appeared in small squares across my screen. All but one were women, and I was the youngest by far. We went round one by one, explaining our situation. My quivering nerves settled as I heard each person speak. Until then, I'd been alone in unfamiliar territory, but that call felt like the beginnings of a map, hearing about similar predicaments that could chart some of the way for me, having the reality of my new daily life witnessed, and witnessed by people who understood it through shared experience. Deirdre joined a couple of weeks after I did. Her husband's Alzheimer's had deteriorated rapidly in the preceding months. Although she had three adult children, they all lived far away and worked full-time, rarely finding time to visit. Deirdre felt isolated with her husband normally, but this had worsened during the first COVID-19 lockdown. Her mood had plummeted, she told us. She spoke haltingly, explaining that she just couldn't see the point anymore, that she didn't know how to go on, each phrase pushed out with great effort as if countering a natural reticence, her disclosures peppered with apologies and self-reprimands: 'Sorry', 'I don't mean to sound like this', 'I shouldn't moan.' She explained she thought her kids didn't call or visit much because they didn't think of her as being 'alone'. After all, in their minds, she was at home with their dad. But their dad had largely lost his memory and many of his bodily functions. He was no longer her husband, the man with whom she'd built her life over the decades. They were together in their home, but he was lost in it, unsure where he was or who Deirdre was, so that she, too, felt lost.

Sickness and care are alchemists: they take relationships and invert and upturn them, metamorphosing parents into children, children into parents, and lovers into dependants. Tracy clearly struggles with this aspect of caring for her father in Michigan, telling me: 'He does act like a child, and that's hard because he's been my dad, telling me what to do, and here I am trying to communicate with him and [be] someone who has to take care of him, but still be his daughter ... it's just a weird situation.' She thinks it's this kind of thing, and the mental toll it takes on the caregiver, that people who haven't been caregivers don't understand, and so is missed by the outside world: 'I think people think you just go over there, cook a couple of meals.' Perhaps most distressingly for Deirdre, her husband had developed aphasia, a condition that meant he could no longer speak or understand any speech, meaning the shared vocabulary they'd spent thirty years cultivating was added to their tally of losses. When she wasn't talking to us in the weekly support call, she was talking into silence.

I considered all this as I sat beside my mum that evening at the hospital. I thought she'd fallen asleep, but then her voice came.

'It's a shame we don't all live like Coralie, really.'

An answer from an unexpected place

Coralie was my great-aunt, a Catholic nun born in 1922. She'd died a few years earlier, and had appeared in my life only a handful of times: a willowy, stern-seeming lady with high cheekbones and pepper-coloured hair. Two generations later, I'd never considered that Coralie's life might have relevant wisdom to offer. But that night at the hospital, before the ward sister kicked me out for the evening, my mum told me a little family secret. Many years before, after a visit to London, she'd driven Coralie back home to the coastal town where she lived. It was a long drive, and the two women had discussed their lives. My mum's relationship with her then-partner had recently broken down and she was at the end of her tether with the trials and tribulations of love. She didn't expect a sympathetic ear from Coralie; she was a divorced single mum exiting yet another relationship, speaking to a Catholic nun. But unexpectedly, Coralie divulged that she understood all too well the wish to avoid the complexities of life and love. She hadn't become a nun purely out of piety, as everyone assumed. As the eldest daughter of six children during the 1930s, she felt she'd been tasked with an unfair share of domestic drudgery in her upbringing, and she didn't want the same to be true in her adulthood. She'd become a nun partly through faith, but also because she wanted to avoid the traditional family life that had belaboured her youth. As an Ursuline nun, she found a happy hybrid of independence and community, embedded in a broad and reliable network of care – a kind of 'family by choice'.

This was why my mum was thinking of Coralie late that night, as she and I worried quietly about how we'd cope with her care once she was discharged. Coralie had a community of nuns around her always – from her early days as a novice in the convent, to her time spent living in a shared church-owned house while she worked in an east London parish, to the order's nursing home by the sea, where she lived out her final days, and where sisters would pop into her room to suggest answers to her beloved crosswords. In a community like this, care was spread over many shoulders, so nobody had to worry about having enough kin on whom to rely, and no caregiver was relegated to the isolated and difficult existence that I, Deirdre, and millions of others shared.

This made me wonder if Coralie's story might contain a wiser approach to care than the current crisis-ridden situation. I'm not suggesting we all become Ursuline nuns, but Coralie's commitment to the church resulted in a network of care in her old age that did not degrade or dehumanise, nor put undue strain on a lone individual, but instead was part and parcel of the community in which she'd spent her life. It was as if, by living within that community, the idea of 'kin' had shifted from a noun, something static and fixed, defined by biology or law, and become a verb, 'kinning', the ongoing creation of family beyond conventional bounds.

Kirsty Woodard has worked on eldercare issues for years, but it wasn't until she realised she wasn't going to have children of her own that she noticed an enormous and overlooked problem in that field: the growing number of adults without children. Around one in five people born in 1967 didn't have children at the end of their childbearing years, compared with one in nine of the generation before them. The United Nations estimates that half of the world's population is living in countries with below-replacement levels of fertility.[3] In Japan, the birth rate reached an all-time low in 2019, dipping below 900,000 births for the first time since governments began tracking it in 1899.[4] In the USA, the number of people needing care is expected to outstrip family members available to provide it by seventy-one per cent by 2050.[5]

Women 'failing' to have children is a much-discussed topic in the media, yet the implications of this for eldercare have yet to make an impact on how we think about and arrange ourselves as human beings with needs.

'Because we've talked a lot, haven't we?' Kirsty says animatedly when we speak via Zoom. 'We, the society, have talked a lot about all these women not having children and all of that . . . in various ways, in ways of shaming and in ways of celebrating . . . but like so much with women, once you get past the age of forty-five, you become invisible anyway. And it was like, what do you think happens or will happen to all these women who don't have children? And when I spoke to people that I worked with in the age sector in various different organisations and said, "Has this ever come up?", they all said, "No, it has never come up as an issue. It's never been raised as an issue. We've never thought about it." Kirsty is so passionate about it that she's worked on the topic for five years unpaid, determined to get it into the spotlight and start designing solutions.

And, of course, the formations in which we live have changed, so even when people do have children and other relatives, they're likely to be more geographically dispersed. Throughout the twentieth century, the phenomenon of the biological and legal family living together or in proximity has generally declined across the West. In *Family and Kinship in East London*, a seminal 1957 sociological study, a lively account is given of the ways in which geographical proximity created strong family caregiving networks around the bustling streets. More than half of the women whom the study surveyed had seen their mothers within the last twenty-four hours, and over eighty per cent within the last week. How many of us can say the same? In that era, around one third to one half of elderly people in the UK lived in a house with one of their children; by the 1990s, this had dropped to fifteen per cent at most.[6] In the last decade, multigenerational living has increased in both the US and the UK, but this is largely because of adult children living with their parents due to economic constraints, rather than because of care considerations. The COVID-19 pandemic might change this: 'granny units' have been described by *Forbes* as 'all the rage'[7] as nursing-home deaths make families prefer home-based care. We'll have to see whether this trend lasts.

Even if the family were restabilised, not everyone will have a family of bio-legal kin, meaning the conventional familial ties of biology, marriage or adoption. As Woodard's important work points out, there must be more imaginative structures in place. It's intriguing – not to mention worrying and frustrating – that while we seem capable of recognising that technology reshapes the world, that politics goes through eras, revolutions and revivals, and that belief systems can weaken or radicalise, the family is still taken as sacrosanct, an ideal that we either inhabit or seek to reach, rather than something archaic, outrun by changes and advances that require us to rethink the very concept.

As our populations age, we must start to prepare solutions or face a catastrophe when it comes to the bodies of our loved ones – and also our own. We must confront the frailty of the family and create new ideas that provide sustainable care without generating the kind of strain experienced by Deirdre, me and so many others. We can do this by moving away from the family and instead broadening our conception of kinship. Historic and contemporary movements that have created forms of 'families of choice' can provide us with inspiration. These movements generate what sociologists call 'fictive kin': that is, kin selected voluntarily outside conventional ties. They are examples of kinning in action.

My great-aunt Coralie found fictive kin in the Ursuline order of Catholic nuns. By seeking family in a community of the like-minded, she was a descendant of an oft-forgotten feminist movement of the Middle Ages. The medieval 'beguine' phenomenon involved many thousands of women across Europe, especially in Belgium, renouncing the expectations of a normal life and marriage, and living together as 'lay nuns' – that is, as deeply religious women, but without taking church vows or living on church property. Beguines would slowly buy houses near each other, taking over spaces in cities and turning them into 'beguinages', complexes where they lived together according to their own sets of rules. In Belgium alone, there were 111 beguinages, and their populations ranged from a handful of beguines to hundreds and, occasionally, thousands. Like Coralie, the beguines found in religion a vehicle to avoid the family, while still being able to practise kinning. And these communities were very much orientated towards care. According to Laura Swan, author of *The Wisdom of the Beguines: The Forgotten Story of a Medieval Women's Movement*, 'beguines pooled their resources in order to serve the sick and destitute by building and operating infirmaries and alms-houses'. They were known especially for tending to lepers and for providing palliative care. At times, their infirmaries were also used to support poor women and children. Care was also available for the beguines themselves; once a woman had been a beguine for four years, 'she could be considered for support by, or admittance to, the infirmary if and when needed'.

Some scholars attribute the surprising size and attraction of the movement to changes in marital patterns taking place throughout that period. This was the emergence of the northern 'European Marriage Pattern', a term coined by Hungarian-British academic John Hajnal in 1965. This pattern entailed households headed by a husband and wife of similar ages who entered marriage later in life than southern European counterparts, where the bride was conventionally considerably younger than the husband and marriages took place at a younger age overall. In the northern European pattern, the couple married when they were capable of being financially independent from their parents and could set up a separate household. Compared to southern Europeans, they also had fewer children.[8] This established the 'nuclear family' and loosened previously strong extended networks. The historian Peter Laslett explains that this led to 'nuclear family hardship', referring to the difficulties generated by living in these atomised units rather than remaining in parental households and extending the family from that base.[9] This shift in kinship structures curtailed women's potential communities of care and, if they didn't marry, left them in a highly vulnerable situation.[10] Becoming a beguine, by contrast, afforded women the security of knowing they would be cared for when needed.

Oppression and social exclusion can drive the impetus for fictive kin. This is no less true for LGBTQ communities than it was for the women of the patriarchal Middle Ages. Rejection by the family, combined with the care requirements wrought by AIDS, has historically led LGBTQ people to seek out chosen kin, constructing their own families of choice to provide security and support. The 1995 collection of essays, *Friends and Lovers: Gay Men Write about the Families They Create*, sought to explore the nature of these chosen families for gay men. Their writings describe deep and important bonds of equal meaning to the bio-legal family ties that they replaced. They also serve to reveal the poverty of our language when it comes to siting care outside the family. When John tries to encapsulate the role that his close friend, Tom, plays in his life, he explains that: 'It has finally come into our vocabulary that Tom is my significant other.' It's taken eight years for them to use that term, even though Tom cares for John most days and does everything from buying groceries to helping him dress in the mornings.

So deep is the trust between the two men that Tom has John's power of attorney, investing in Tom the right to take legal and medical decisions on his behalf. The bond and intimacy of the daily shared life John describes is commonly expected in romantic relationships – in marriages – yet Tom and John are not romantically or sexually involved. Calling on us to find a more meaningful vocabulary for such arrangements, John warns that 'to call us merely best friends denies the depth of who we are to each other'. Outside the language of 'mere' friendship or sexual intimacy, we lack labels for many crucial caring relationships. As professor of sociology Anna Muraco has opined, 'There is no sufficient social script to guide or characterise non-biological, platonic, emotionally intimate and socially reliant relationships between friends.'[11] And yet, the trends described earlier require us to start developing wider notions of family so that we can secure the care we need.

The examples given so far focus on communities of people who've been subject to social exclusion or oppression due to identity characteristics – namely, being female and being LGBTQ.

In her work on fictive kin, Muraco points out that 'in general, non-marginalised straight people who have access to nuclear families are not expected to rely upon chosen family bonds'; fictive kin are presumed to be a kind of second-best, sought out only when our bio-legal relations are strained or falling short in some way. Yet this cultural assumption makes us miss out on potential bonds that could be life-sustaining in times of need. Coralie's faith legitimised the swapping of a biological family for an unrelated one, but why do we need gods or oppression to legitimise these choices?

Inspired by Coralie's example, a year into my mum's illness, I set up a women's circle – a group of friends who came together once a month to discuss topics of interest, eat together and grow our bond. I knew most of them already, but carving out a deliberate and regular space to meet and to share our experiences and worries strengthened our relationships. It was the one social event I tried to make sure happened amidst the chaos of my caregiving life. A few months after I'd begun the circle, I found myself in an east London emergency department with a high fever and difficulty breathing. When the hospital receptionist asked me for my next-of-kin's contact details, I immediately welled up. I suddenly realised I couldn't say my mum anymore. She couldn't travel or care for me – and besides, I didn't think the hospital would be too impressed if the person I dragged to the emergency department was very evidently bald from cancer treatment. I gaped at the woman, heaving in each breath and trying not to seem mad for becoming upset by the question. Then I gave her the name and number of one of the women in the circle.

Sophia turned up about forty minutes later, waited with me while the doctors confirmed I had pneumonia, and then came home with me, where she frowned and muttered at my messy bedroom and plied me with madeleines and cups of tea. Without those monthly meetings we'd shared, I doubt I'd have had the courage to give Sophia's name – or that of any friend. My socialised politeness would have sought to avoid suddenly impinging on their plans. Its synonymity with 'home' means it comes imbued with ideals of shelter, warmth and safety. In poet Robert Frost's words: 'Home is the place where, when you have to go there, they have to take you in.' Of course, none of this is true universally. The family is as often a site of violence and abuse as it is one of safety and love. But even when it's the latter, there's a shadow side that goes unseen. Being able to be safe and warm *inside* the family means there is, inevitably, an *outside*. When we consider the family as the place in which we should all seek care, and furthermore, as the *correct* port of call for that care, we inevitably exclude those who lack family from crucial care. Even if we have a family ourselves, we make it much harder to reach out beyond the private realm when we need help. In their 1982 book *The Antisocial Family*, Professors Michèle Barrett and Mary Mcintosh describe this shadow side of the family, and are worth quoting in full:

> 'It is as if the family had drawn comfort and security into itself and left the outside world bereft. As a bastion against a bleak society it has made that society bleak. It is indeed a major agency for caring, but in monopolising care it has made it harder to undertake other forms of care. It is indeed a unit of sharing, but

in demanding sharing within it has made other relations tend to become more mercenary. It is indeed a place of intimacy, but in privileging the intimacy of close kin it has made the outside world cold and friendless, and made it harder to sustain relations of security and trust except with kin. Caring, sharing and loving would be more widespread if the family did not claim them for its own.'[12]

The regularity, structure and commitment of our monthly women's circle meetings had subverted this insider/outsider idea of family, in its own small way. We half-jokingly referred to ourselves as 'the sisterhood', a pleasing evocation of Coralie and her Ursulines. We had created a burgeoning sense of duty and responsibility to one another, entering the beginning stages of kinning. At that time, I lived in a very rundown house in east London. One of the kitchen window panes was cracked, and through it, a pale green tendril from the garden had begun to grow. I liked to think of the women's circle as like that exploratory stalk; we were wending our way through the boundaries established by conventional notions of family, gently introducing to ourselves the idea that we might outgrow and overcome them to create something more expansive and supportive. Michael Rowe, another essayist in *Friends and Lovers: Gay Men Write about the Families They Create*, writes that he has 'made brothers out of my two oldest friends'. When one of his 'brothers' had a son, he became Uncle Michael, and says that for him, that child is the next generation of his family, despite there being no blood or legal tie. He is uncertain where the line between friendship and brotherhood is drawn and crossed, 'but it has to do with trust and time'. He has cultivated a different kind of brotherhood, using these ingredients, just as my sisterhood and I had been doing. For him, and for me and the women in my circle, these bonds provide something we lack elsewhere, and may in time come to provide us with care that would otherwise be absent.

Despite the importance of these relationships in our lives, we don't talk about and value them in the way that we need to if we're to meet the requirements of care. We might consider them 'disenfranchised kin', in the sense that these kinship structures exist but are ignored, overlooked and shut out. In 2004, social scientists Sasha Roseneil and Shelley Budgeon sought to explore these 'cultures of intimacy and care' by interviewing adults who weren't living with a partner. They deemed that these were the people most likely to have constructed alternative forms of kinship. And they were right: their research uncovered stories in which people became each other's kin by choice, providing care outside conventional labels. One interviewee, Dale, was a forty-nine-year-old man with a range of friends, neighbours and ex-partners whom he defined as his 'kinship network' and who had been crucial in providing care. A serious motorbike accident had hospitalised him for the best part of two years; during that period, these chosen kin were a vital support, even looking after his mother when he was unable to help her. Another interviewee, Eleanor, was diagnosed with cancer: her 'family by choice' rallied around, attending hospital tests with her and running a sleepover rota so that they could 'share collectively in the needed provision of care'. Dale, Eleanor and other interviewees are creating 'generalised reciprocity', a core characteristic of kinning. Generalised reciprocity occurs when the giving of gifts, services, or anything really, takes place without an immediate expectation of something in return. It's crucial for caregiving, which requires us to perform tasks and services for loved ones without that expectation, and indeed with the possibility of never getting anything 'in return'. The people Roseneil and Budgeon identified, and the examples found in many other studies of fictive kin, have made it clear that relationships beyond the traditional family can involve this kind of reciprocity, and that they can be a crucial part of caregiving – as important as family, and sometimes more so.

The COVID-19 pandemic ought to have awoken us to aspects of this. In two ways, many people discovered that their conventional family weren't the people on whom they relied. First, those living in house shares with friends or acquaintances were forced to recognise a deep and intimate interdependency usually only assigned to bio-legal kin, even if they're countries away. Second, many people – especially families – were acutely aware that their family was in fact a constituent part of a broader network of care, one that needed to 'bubble' with other people to share childcare or eldercare, or simply for company. If we think again of Coralie, her life was constructed in a way that meant this idea of a care network wasn't a surprise. Despite her childlessness, she had a community built into the fabric of her life. As a nun, the traditional family was unavailable to her. And rather than being a loss, through the lens of care, this was a gift.

When I think of Deirdre and me, on those video calls, I see us trapped on lonely islands of care, brought together only through our computer screens. Most of us aired frustrations with family members, their absence or seeming lack of commitment to the situation. Clearly, we held some sort of idea that familial care was a duty, but one that many shirked. The solution to this doesn't lie with either government-provided care or privately paid care. Both those sources of care can alleviate the amount of work done by a lone caregiver and provide for acute situations that need specialist support, but neither is a sufficient replacement (without institutionalising the person needing care), because, as we've already established, someone must be there between the shifts, arranging and overseeing things, and so on. Some people who need care also refuse 'outside' sources. One study examining caregiving relationships between neighbours and frail elderly people found that in some of those instances, the latter had refused government-provided care – indeed, sometimes lying to avoid being earmarked as someone in need of it – so there was no (moral) alternative but to step in and support them.[13] My mother repeatedly refused hired care workers, despite my evident strain. She didn't want strangers around the house, a sentiment with which many people concur. To some extent, the idea of fictive kin can change this lonely landscape of care, conjoining islands as we learn the practice of kinning, spreading the care load across more shoulders.

Meeting the women at the vanguard

On a hot day in June 2021, I took a train and a bus from my London neighbourhood further north to find out about a different and better way of living. It wasn't supposed to be an especially warm day, but the English weather likes to surprise, and I was glad I'd chanced bare limbs as I sweated towards my destination. This journey was precious to me. Since my conversation with my mother about Coralie, I'd been voraciously researching ways of living in community. It had brought me to the Older Women's Co-Housing (OWCH) project, happily located in the same city as me, and I was on my way there, feeling my mum's presence with me, though she'd died months previously. From the outside, OWCH (pronounced 'ouch') looks like a normal, stylishly designed new complex of apartments. The estate itself, named 'New Ground' due to its pioneering spirit, took years to plan and finally came into being in 2016 in a leafy area of Barnet, north London. Twenty-five brick apartments with handsome dark grey balconies overlook a shared central lawn with private gardens around its edge. There's also a shared 'co-house' for communal gatherings, such as the weekly meal together, an occasional film club or meetings about running OWCH in general. The project has received a slew of awards for its design and architecture. I was welcomed at the door by Maria Brenton, a charismatic expert on co-housing who supported OWCH to its realisation. We sat together with residents Jude and Charlotte, having tea and chit-chatting as I marvelled at the lovely gardens and learned about their way of life.

The history of co-housing is rich, but hopefully poor in comparison to its future. Unlike communes or shared houses, where everyone lives in the same home, co-housing is a blend of private dwellings with shared spaces, amenities and governance. In 1987, a group of nine single older women in Denmark established the first older people's co-housing arrangement, called Midgården. They took over a five-storey apartment block, turning the ground floor into common areas and the remainder into individual private dwellings. Their example spawned a movement; by 2000, there were over 100 such schemes across Denmark, and more in Sweden, the Netherlands, Germany, USA and beyond.

In Montreuil, France, a group of older women share OWCH's proclivity for punchy names, having created their own co-housing arrangement called La Maison des Babayagas, or 'The House of Witches'. The scheme was spearheaded by feminist activist Thérèse Clerc, who, like me, began thinking about different ways of living after the death of her mother in the mid-1990s. Born in 1927, she spent her life fighting for women's rights, focusing first on the right to abortion and contraception, and later establishing a refuge in Montreuil for women who had been victims of gender-based violence. Her concomitant experience of caring for her bedridden mother inspired her to try to arrange a different kind of old age for herself, one in which women could 'grow old together as independent, free and useful citizens'.[14] Today, La Maison des Babayagas is a thriving institution on Rue de la Convention, comprising a six-storey building with twenty-one apartments for women aged over sixty. It fulfils Clerc's dream of creating an enriching and collective life for older women; in 2019 alone, its residents enjoyed a film club, ran an art exhibition that raised money for its ongoing cultural and horticultural pursuits, and hosted debates on political issues.

Co-housing allows people to choose a group with whom to live in proximity, sharing space and facilities that they collectively determine and control, while still having their own private home. In some cases in the US, a coordinator is appointed who ensures caring needs are met. However, unlike in many retirement villages or care homes, these needs are met by other community members, not outsourced to paid workers.[15] This is a world away from the sheltered housing in which many elderly and frail across the world find themselves living, where they don't have control over the resources they use nor the general management of the complex or services, and are likely to be cared for by paid workers with whom they may lack a rapport. This isn't to say that members are each other's caregivers, per se. The women of OWCH are clear that they aren't and won't be. Their policy on the subject is: 'The group undertakes "to look out for rather than look after each other". Where an individual has care needs, she is expected to have arrangements in place to meet them.'[16] While this creates a clear requirement for people who have acute care needs, I suspect it's also a product of what we think when we hear the words 'caregiver' or 'care'. Circumscribed within narrow concepts of the family, it comes to mean someone who does everything, often to the general detriment of their own life, and who is probably very overwhelmed and stressed. It's a concept that is also highly medicalised, thanks to the global trend for reducing the length of hospital stays. But probing further, the OWCH way of living means that a lot of caregiving does take place. 'We have health buddies,' Charlotte tells me. She and the neighbouring women on each side of her have each other's house keys and family contacts, and she says: 'If anything's needed in the middle of the night, I

147

would know without hesitation I could ring [their] doorbells . . . it's like having this extra layer of support.' When Jude broke her arm, this way of living meant that there wasn't only one person who helped her, but many, and sometimes they've done rotas to provide sufficient support to one another. The shared resources of OWCH aren't only the common house or the central lawn, but also these acts of care.

Relationships and shared resources like those cultivated at New Ground and La Maison des Babayagas, or researched by Roseneil and Budgeon, don't fit into the traditional idea of the family. This disenfranchisement obscures those families of choice that already exist and prevents us from being imaginative about creating more of these types of systems and relationships. We can see their exclusion when we examine bureaucratic forms that enquire about our relationships. On UK tax self-assessment forms, you can select your 'relationship status' from a range of categories: married, widowed, divorced, single or cohabiting. But how might many of the people we've met in this chapter respond to that question? What is the relationship between John and Tom, for instance? Tom is a platonic, non-cohabiting significant other – where does he fit? What of the women of New Ground, La Maison des Babayagas, or the many and growing number of comparable communities around the world? Censuses reveal these biases too. The UK census asks: 'Who usually lives at your address?' Respondents can tick clear categories, such as 'family members', 'students who live away from home during termtime', 'housemates, tenants or lodgers'. This disaggregation clearly sep-arates the idea of the traditional family from that of 'others', who might only be 'housemates, tenants or lodgers'. It also presumes that people live in a manner that has neatly circumscribable boundaries based on a single abode. Who does Jude live with in her apartment at OWCH? We could say she lives there alone, because she doesn't share her apartment with anyone, but does she really *live alone*? Why are we so focused on who lives in our houses? Later in the census, it asks how members of the household are related to each other. Twelve options are given, such as husband, wife, stepchild, grandchild, and then a thirteenth, which is merely 'unrelated'. The USA's census follows a similar pattern, with 'other non-relative' the paltry description afforded to those you might live with but not be related to by blood, marriage or romance.

It's clear in the way these questions are phrased that we have no word for the kinds of bonds created through fictive kin, and no spaces for projects and systems that might constitute kinning. No wonder we think the silver bullet must lie outside us, with either the government or the market. Cultures other than white British or European American families are useful to consider here, as some have deeply embedded social structures that rely on what we might call 'unrelated relations'. In the Mexican community, whether in Mexico itself or in the diaspora, there is a firmly established culture of *compadrazgo,* or 'co-parenthood'. *Compadres* (co-fathers) and *comadres* (co-mothers) play an important and intimate role in family life. Likewise, African and African-American communities have firmly embedded forms of fictive kin. Historical slavery led to many Africans losing ties with their blood kin, causing a practice of replacing absent families with fictive kin from the same ethnic or national community.[17] 'Othermothers' are commonly found in African-American communities. An 'othermother' is a woman with no biological ties to the family unit who is 'functioning within the parameters of a biological maternal figure . . . with expectations of obligation equal to those of blood-relatives'. These women play a hugely important role in the lives of their 'children', and yet our standard approaches to families leave them out of the picture.

The US National Black Nurses Association, in collaboration with academics, has sought to remedy this by calling for a way to capture information about African-American patients' fictive kin. This is because family – fictive or otherwise – plays a vital role in the prevention of many diseases, such as diabetes and heart disease, by encouraging lifestyle changes, screenings and similar interventions. It's common practice in medicine to capture data about a person's traditional family, but not about those people whom they might consider family but don't fit within those narrow parameters.[18] Similarly, Professor Maryalice Jordan-Marsh of the University of Southern California has noted her concern that 'there is little documentation on the extent to which fictive kin participate in interactions with the healthcare system, such as accompanying older adults on visits, contributing to decision-making, or providing direct care . . . The nursing literature is remarkably bereft of references to extended "family" that are not related by marriage or genetics.' This is despite, she goes on to say, the fact that fictive kin are 'potentially economical, family-friendly solutions to the burgeoning social problem of caring for an increasingly diverse, often frail, older adult population with few surviving and willing family caregivers'. Without capturing these kinds of important relationships in our societies, we can't fully understand caregiving – either its current reality or, even more crucially, its potential future.

Blind spots are also found in law, creating confusion and diminishing care in tangible ways. In 2012, Canada's *Globe and Mail* newspaper reported on the deportation of a seventy-three-year-old American woman. Ms Inferrera had been living in Canada for decades and, since her Canadian friend Ms Sanford's husband died, had been living with her and providing care for her, as Ms Sanford suffered from both a heart condition and dementia. Despite this crucial caregiving role, Ms Inferrera's application for residency was denied. Thankfully, public outcry at the separation of the two women saw Canada relent and Ms Inferrera safely returned to her friend's side, but the case demonstrates that the role of the chosen kin in caregiving is missing from legal protections. Professor of philosophy Elizabeth Brake of Rice University said: 'These two women were not romantically involved, and so, presumably, did not consider marriage an option. Why should their relationship lack recognition and support because they are "just" friends – friends who have cohabited for decades and cared for one another materially?'[19]

Caregiving requires social bonds and proximity. Both these facets have long been assumed to reside within the traditional family. In many cases today, they still do. But increasing numbers of people needing care, and people providing it, are alone and without sufficient familial support. The future seems bleak if we continue to centre caregiving on the enfeebled family. To prepare appropriately for the future of care, we must leave behind the traditional family and learn the practice of kinning, building families of choice that are more expansive, imaginative and robust.

What might have been

In this kind of radically imagined future, Deirdre might have a range of chosen family members cultivated over the course of her life who have no blood or romantic tie to her, but who participate in the reciprocity of familial relations, and who can become part of the support system in place for her husband. The absence of her own children becomes irrelevant, because ideas about who is and who is not officially 'family' have changed. Or perhaps my mum could have been living in co-housing with fellow seniors, and would never have had to speak that strangled and fearful question: *What are we going to do?* My response to her question that night at the hospital was stuttering and uncertain. Sometimes, answers come too late in life, and they did for my mum's care. If I'd understood Coralie's choice when I was younger, if I'd learned about the beguines and the incredible older women's co-housing schemes, perhaps my expanded imagination could have brought practical change into our lives. As I kissed my mum on the forehead before I left the hospital for the night, I didn't realise I had the seeds of a solution taking root in my mind. It would take me many, many months of reading and investigating to understand what these seeds were, how pioneers in history and today have made them grow, and what an updated version of kinship might look like, one that provides a stronger base for care. For my mum, those seeds never got the chance to grow; they can only flourish in my imagination now. I like to imagine her there though, in a different final chapter to her life, without the isolation and the strain felt by both of us. She's content, in a lovingly decorated flat above a communal ground floor, her window overlooking a verdant courtyard. I'm there too, but the furrow in my forehead is smoothed. When I kiss her as I leave, both she and I are smiling, confident that a dozen wise old women are ready to lend a hand until I return.

CHAPTER 5

On the Mind:
Confronting a Convenient Stigma

'We are discontinuous beings, individuals who perish in isolation in the midst of an incomprehensible adventure . . .'

– Georges Bataille[1]

In late summer 2018, I lay in bed, listening to a scratching, scuffling sound that was far too close for comfort. The next-door neighbours had done some building work, which had dislodged a rat from its usual abode. It was now stuck between our walls. I knew this because when the scratching and scuffling had begun a few days before, I'd moved gingerly over to its location, ready to jump fast on to my bed if anything emerged. There was a sliver of a gap between the floorboards and the skirting; in that crack, a pink, rubbery tail flicked about in a trapped frenzy.

I'm not phobic of rats, but I certainly don't like them, nor do

Who Cares

I want them in my bedroom, trapped or otherwise. I put gaffer tape along the crack, making it even less likely the rat would creep into my room, then slept fitfully, listening guiltily to its derangement, my duvet tucked tightly around my body as protection. I knew it wasn't normal to coexist with the rodent like that, but I didn't have the energy to do more. I was exhausted and ill. I'd been accompanying my mum to hospital trips twice a week – one for chemo, one for tests to monitor her. She needed a cannula in her arm for the chemo, which she hated because doctors always struggled to find a viable vein. I left each appointment drained from trying to soothe her. This was alongside my job and, on top of both, I had a virus I couldn't shake. I needed help or a break, something to let me get well and find the strength to deal with the small trials of daily life, which had become beyond me.

I'd been with my boyfriend for a few months by then. He had dark curls and green eyes, a strong nose and stronger shoulders. I thought it was miraculous that he'd fallen in love with me at the same moment that my mum got diagnosed: something light in a darkening world. Her illness was simultaneously invisible in our relationship and its articulation, like the negative space around an object. On the surface, we lived a conventional young-ish couple's life. We made large brunches together on Sunday mornings (before I went to the hospital), or hung out with friends (while I kept my phone on loud in case she had an emergency). At cinemas and clubs and cafés, I'd listen to him while silently thinking through the logistics of the week ahead, remembering I needed to count her remaining pills in case she was close to running out, or wondering whether to risk her ire and tell the doctor she still wasn't drinking enough water. When we talked about politics and all the things that needed changing in our world, he'd speak with a youthful fire that had such vigorous energy, it astonished me. Not because I couldn't fathom being that way, but because I knew that I had once been like that myself, truly in the realm of the living, and that now my vitality had been sapped out of me. I brought dragging, tired fears with me everywhere I went, surviving in between our dates on toast and slivers of dwindling hope. So it was in this context that he came to stay, on the third night of the scratching-scuffling. I had warned him about it, but perhaps he hadn't understood, because he was disgusted by the situation and angry about it limiting his sleep. In the morning, he told me he wouldn't stay again until the rat was gone. He left for work. I lay there, wondering what to do, feverish, with aches in my limbs from the virus, a dizziness when I stood, a sinking feeling that I could disintegrate entirely and nobody would notice until I was nothing but dust.

Then, around three months later, on a cold and dry November evening, we were on a journey across London. We'd been away for a weekend in Ireland and were supposed to divide at a point equidistant from his home and from my mother's in Greenwich. I was moving in with her for a while because she'd just been discharged from hospital after a risky stem-cell transplant. My backpack was hot pink. I'd bought it only a fortnight earlier, an attempt to inject light-heartedness into life, to demonstrate to him that I could still be fun, even though I was brittle and anxious constantly. Unsurprisingly, the weekend hadn't gone well. In the cavernous lobby of London Bridge station, with my ridiculous pink backpack digging into my shoulders, he ended our relationship. My memories of what happened next are confused: a clutching, begging motion; a pleading, pushing, whining voice that surely couldn't be mine? A fog all around me where there'd been station architecture only moments before; a black shadow splitting me open from my skull to the pockmarked floor. It hadn't been the plan, but I think because of my near-total disassembly, he took me all the way to Greenwich. I wondered why he was so keen to get me there, into my mother's house, as if there was anything inside it other than more pain, more grief. There must have been people all around us on the train, but I couldn't see them. Only him, and the strange sensations of my joints slipping apart and slapping back together as if I'd been soul-switched with a broken puppet. I can recall little of what he said, other than that he loved me, but it was too hard. It *was* too hard, I thought, between desperate pleas. At Greenwich, we sat on the stone ledge that overlooks the Thames, watching the black waves of the river shining like an oil slick. I hoped my heart would stop beating so that I didn't have to keep dragging myself through time that was so heavy and thick.

Eventually he got me, staggeringly, to my mother's front doorstep. I was already an hour late, completely irresponsible because she was in a high-risk state. There was no safe harbour for me anywhere – him in front of me, his beautiful face firm at the mouth with its decision; her inside, red-eyed and wavering in her mortality. I tried clutching at him one more time and he stepped backwards, both arms out, palms up, as if keeping me at bay, his face curving into the mask of distaste that he'd used when he left my bedroom that morning in late summer. I got into my mum's house, did what she needed and went to my room, then spent the night retching and shivering and failing to sleep. There was no scratching-scuffling in that bedroom, but I felt a rat was there all the same. It was me. I had become a pestilent, discarded thing. Something from which to walk away at a relieved and disgusted speed.

I understand now what happened to me in that phase of life. I experienced what many caregivers do: a mental breakdown, the slow kind, like a lobster in a pot that no one notices until it's screaming. Mental illness wasn't new to me – depression and related issues had stalked me all my life – but I'd been well for a long time. With hindsight, it was unsurprising that my situation would make these issues recur. It's been a comfort to realise I'm not the only one who's been broken by care. Ayesha in Kathmandu also knows its shattering power all too well. After her mother died, she tells me:

> I had a complete meltdown . . . it hit me and I was very, very broken, and it affected my relationship. I broke up with my partner. We were thinking of a future together, potentially, but I didn't know who I was anymore, because I felt so broken and like I didn't have anything to give . . . I don't think it was a justified move on my part. I just didn't have anything left in me to explain why I was acting the way I was, why I was feeling the way I was. I was completely bogged down by years of emotions. And I mean, I was, I would say, really depressed . . . I just wanted to curl up in a ball and not wake up, because life was

just so . . . so meaningless.

Since her mother died, Ayesha has suffered a brain aneurysm. 'They think it might be stress,' she told me.

So common is psychological breakdown for caregivers that the term 'caregiver stress syndrome' has been coined. Those three words are a hygienic way of describing the debris of lives that could have been different, hearts that take years to put back together, mosaics of what they once were. I know now that I couldn't deal with the rat, and my immune system couldn't keep me well, because I was a hundred miles beyond burnout, and I desperately needed help. I'd been suffering from panic attacks, night terrors and general anxiety. I'd started to have a sensation like a sudden surge of electricity in my brain, something known as 'brain zaps' that can be caused by extreme stress. The noises of the tube on my commute to work felt like pneumatic drills clattering in my head, despite it being a soundtrack that had accompanied my whole adult life. I was behaving in odd and unregulated ways. I know too, as we'll see in this chapter, that aside from the obvious difficulties of being in a relationship with someone behaving in those ways, my proximity to sickness and death will also have been offputting for evolutionary reasons. But back then, I didn't know any of that. I was just lost in grief and pain, required to go to work, to care for her, and to pretend I still lived in the same world as everyone else. And I failed.

The Charybdis of caregiving

'There is no future and the present is so miserable.' [2]

'I'm absolutely shattered . . . I've asked the [doctor] for sleeping pills, but he just told me to jog on. At least if I could rest, I wouldn't feel so miserable all the time.' [3]

'I can't do it anymore, and there is no help or way out.'[4]

As these posts show, spending time on caregiver forums is to enter a Charybdis of misery and desperation. As we know from Chapter 1, caregivers are more likely to suffer from depression and anxiety than the general public. 'Even being in the [eldercare] business,' Karen tells me, 'I never anticipated it would feel this bad. It doesn't feel like when I was caring for an infant. I had joy when I was caring for my babies. This isn't joyful at all.'

While most studies on burnout have pertained to occu-pational settings, there's now recognition that kin caregivers experience it too. They can also fall prey to 'compassion fatigue', a specific difficulty that arises when you have empathy for a person or people and must continually witness their suffering without sufficient support or respite. It's been described as 'a heavy heart, a debilitating weariness brought about by repetitive, empathic responses to pain and suffering in others', or 'a physical and spiritual fatigue, or exhaustion that takes over a care-giver'.[5] Symptoms include nightmares, anxiety, sleep problems, hypervigilance, dread of work, absenteeism, errors in judgement, emotional numbness, religious doubts and difficulty concentrating. It sounds familiar. A woman posting online about her experience helping her father to care for her mother encapsulates the kind of complex, guilt-ridden compassion fatigue with which caregivers contend:

> I feel my future cannot start until my mum dies . . . This fills me with despair and then guilt . . . I often wish I would die so I don't have to face this indeterminate period of time when my life is hijacked by my mum's illness . . . I have lost my compassion and resent and hate her . . . guilt plays a huge part in my life now.[6]

Caregivers may be even more prone to both burnout and compassion fatigue than paid workers because they can't escape their 'work'. Research has found that having multiple roles within a job can protect against burnout because people can have some sense of control and choice about their clients and how or when they do tasks. In the study that found this, one professional counsellor explained: 'If I did only this work, I would be bored out of [my] mind . . . It has nothing to do with the people I see; it's about having to empty yourself out so constantly and regularly . . . that wouldn't be healthy, it just wouldn't be healthy.'[7] To some extent, caregivers can choose the order of some of our tasks, but we cannot choose our 'clients', nor can we refuse to do tasks because we consider them to be outside our job descriptions.

The same study found that professionals can protect themselves by 'maintaining a balance between their personal and professional lives'. But what about when it *is* your personal life?

'I don't think I slept for five months,' Ayesha tells me. 'I think the only breaks I took were to shower and to cook meals, but the meals would be for her for the most part, because with all of the medication and the chemo, you lose [your] sense of taste. All the food tastes bad. So it's making seventy different things until she chooses what she likes. So I think everything I did for me somehow involved her in some way or the other . . . I slept on the floor in the same room as her. I didn't even go to my own bedroom.'

In this sort of circumstance, caregivers experience 'role engulfment', a well-chosen term for the feeling that their caregiving role has completely consumed their life. 'Just one last thing,' one forum user writes. 'Does anyone else feel that their own life has been swallowed up and disappeared?'[8]

Unsurprisingly, people who need to care for sick, elderly or impaired loved ones often find their relationships under strain. In the US, eighty per cent of baby boomers caring for an ageing parent say that it's put a strain on their marriage, while forty-six per cent say that it's damaged their romantic relationships. Twenty-five per cent of those who'd divorced say their caring commitments played a 'major role' in that divorce.[9] Articles and problem pages about this abound, with titles like 'My marriage or my mom' and 'Is my marriage over or am I just exhausted from caring for my mum?'[10] Friendships suffer, too. I asked every caregiver I interviewed about their social lives, and all of them described losing friends because of caring, either because of the responsibilities it entails or the discomfort it provokes. Eric in Minnesota, USA had a generous view of this experience:

> There were some really good friends of his [Scott, Eric's husband] that sort of disappeared, and he always wondered why that happened. And I said, 'Honey, there are friends of all different ilks, and ... sometimes you have your good-times friends, you have your bad-times friends, and you have your good-and-bad times friends, and then you have your when-the-shit-hits-the-fan friends, and those can be all different people. Some people just aren't emotionally capable of watching you go through this. They can't bring themselves to do it.'

In recent years, there have been increasing numbers of books, articles and media commentary exposing the harder aspects of motherhood. But there's been no parallel conversation about the deep discomforts of caregiving for the elderly, unwell or impaired. If you care for long enough, and it engulfs your life, you'll probably have thoughts that you wouldn't speak aloud because they're socially unacceptable. You will wish it would end, and soon, even though you know it means losing a loved one. You will resent what it's taking away from you – your time, your energy, your plans for work, love and family. It's a horrible situation, a layer of shame upon a layer of pain.

Without sufficient support, caregivers can snap under the pressure. Griselda Folkard, sixty-nine, and her mother Barbara Innes, 107, lived on Market Street in the quiet town of Builth

Wells, Wales. It would be more accurate to say that Barbara lived in their small flat above the local credit union than in the town itself, because by the time she died in 2013, she hadn't left her bed for fifteen years. Neighbours described Griselda as a quiet and kind person, devoted to caring for her mum. It came as a shock, then, when Griselda and Barbara were reported to have been the oldest ever pair to die in a murder-suicide. Nobody can know precisely why Griselda did what she did, but, in April 2013, she sedated her mother with diazepam and smothered her with a pillow. Afterwards, Griselda ran a bath and drowned herself.

The list of such tragedies is long and indiscriminate of gender, age or place. There's an incongruity in being a caregiver of someone when their condition only worsens, when the sole and inevitable outcome is death. You feel like a bystander at a horrific slow-motion accident, forced to watch and offer paltry aid, but unable to truly help. Is this *care*? At times, it's hard to know what the most caring thing to do would be. Every professional I interviewed for this book had encountered these sorts of thoughts in caregivers, occasional whispers of 'just wishing it was over' and similar. Melanie Goodridge works with the African Caribbean Care Group (ACCG), based in Manchester, UK. When we spoke, she'd encountered a caregiver that very day who'd come into the service feeling suicidal. It's easy to forget that people with one problem may also be navigating others – this woman, on top of her caring role, was navigating immigration issues. 'She'd been here twenty years,' Melanie told me, 'and now they've come for her . . . there's so many seeking asylum now who we could probably help, but they're not allowed to get the help.' Likewise, many elderly people caring for their spouse or impaired adult children are coping with their own medical problems alongside providing care.

Contemporary human culture is afflicted with an ability to identify a problem and prescribe solutions that do nothing to solve its causes. This is especially problematic when political and economic arrangements, shaped by governments, aren't focused on human wellbeing, but on some other goal, be it GDP or the glorification of a leader. In the case of caregiving, there's a plethora of recommended tips to keep your marriage or protect your social life. The study that discovered those stark statistics about baby-boomer caregivers' relationships provides allegedly 'helpful' tips, including: 'Make a concerted effort every day to keep the flame of your love affair with each other alive,' and 'Don't wallow in self-pity; it's a wasted emotion.' Another article purporting to solve caregivers' marital woes recommends remembering to listen to your non-caregiving spouse, and to 'make time for fun and romance together, and make it a top priority'.[11]

While these tips are laughable in their failure to reckon with the deep psychological and physical difficulties faced by care-givers, caregivers themselves report many tactics they use to stay as sane as possible. Eric went running. I ran too, quickly and urgently, and did yoga in quiet moments while my mum slept. Katy enjoys her morning coffee and Ulla loves walks by the river near her home. I'm not from a religious background, but if I was, it's highly likely prayer would have helped me to cope. Studies have found that having religious beliefs or 'spirituality' (defined as the search for the sacred) can make you more likely to experience the positive aspects of caregiving, like having a sense of satisfaction and reward.[12] And various interventions, such as providing caregivers with education about their role, or offering counselling support and the opportunity to connect with others in the same boat, as we've already seen with Carers Worldwide and the WellMed Charitable Foundation, have all been shown to have positive, strain-alleviating effects. These kinds of projects are needed desperately and should be initiated where they don't exist and increased where they do. But we also need to delve deeper to have hope of truly changing the caregivers' psychological experience – which, in case you've forgotten, most likely means your experience too, at some point. To do that, we must leave the personalised interventions to one side and consider the ills of our collective psyche.

Uncomfortable evolutionary truths

When I was in the throes of caregiving, I noticed how people would look uncomfortable or flinch if I raised the topic; how they'd make a sympathetic face followed by flapping gestures, as if they were waving it away, and seemingly for my benefit. One of the most common responses was, 'I couldn't do that.' I've wondered what they meant. I don't think it's literal. If their mother was huddled in bed, quivering and coughing, unable to make herself meals or move without their support, they wouldn't just walk away and leave her there to die. They mean that they don't *want* to do that, and that by believing that we, the caregivers, are somehow super-human and different to them, they'll be spared that Herculean labour. The claim was always delivered as if it was a compliment, obscuring its motivation to keep caregiving at a safe distance.

On group support calls with other caregivers, I heard repeatedly how they felt excluded and abandoned by former friends, how neighbours seemed to hurry away from them as if they were infectious. Line, in Norway, tells me that having Tarjei meant 'we learned which friends to rely on and which friends think it's a nuisance that we are too much work and not flexible enough'. Katy, in England, describes herself as having a 'typical carer's story: I've lost some friends because I wasn't able to go to things and then they just stopped asking. It would still be nice to be asked, even though we both know I'll have to say no. You lose friends.' Safa (not her real name) is eighteen and lives in east London. Since she was twelve, she's been helping to care for her little sister, who has Ehlers-Danlos syndrome, which affects the connective tissue throughout the body, and also Potocki-Lupski syndrome, which Safa describes as meaning she's 'child-minded'. We met in a park café in torrential rain, huddling over hot drinks and hoping we could hear each other over the din of the other customers, the whole park seeking cover simultaneously. When I asked about her friendships, she told me that 'some friends were understanding, others weren't so understanding', and she made a chopping motion as she said she cut the latter group off. They'd make spiteful remarks about her sister, and at first Safa argued with them, but after a while she decided it wasn't worth the energy. Evidently, the loss of friends and people's urge to back away from caregiving situations was an experience common to us all. The reason why lies in our evolution.

Evolutionary psychology seeks to understand our behaviour by considering what function its aspects may have served in our successful adaptation over time. At its worst, it can be considered a reductive approach, trying to explain everything in biological terms, with, presumably, little room to change things so deeply and fundamentally ingrained. At its best, its speculations about why this or that psychological response might have evolved recognises that, while certain responses may have been functional in the past, that doesn't mean they remain so.

Our ancestors faced many threats to their survival. One such threat was disease and infection. Experimental psychology has shown repeatedly, and in many ways, that our aim to avoid disease and infection underlies many of our prejudicial and stigmatising behaviours. This 'disease-avoidance' theory of why some individuals or groups are excluded finds that we developed psychological mechanisms that respond to signs of disease, like rashes or coughing spasms. But this signalling system is over-sensitive. It would have been more costly to make a 'false negative' decision than a 'false positive' one – that is, it would have harmed us more if we'd decided someone's rash was benign and hugged them, only to discover it signified some deadly disease, than to have presumed it was infectious and steered clear, even if it was in fact benign. Our 'disease-avoidance' mechanism is therefore set to a hair trigger; we misapply it repeatedly, ascribing potential contamination more widely than is accurate.[13]

In one experiment, researchers found that people with higher scores of germ-aversion were more likely to associate disabled people with disease.[14] Other experiments have found that people spent more time interacting with others who appeared 'normal' or feigned a temporary physical condition, such as a broken arm, compared to people with more permanent impairments, such as an amputated leg, and also that people stood further away from those described to them as being amputees or epileptics.[15] This aversion extends beyond visible physical impairments or symptoms, too, also applying to objects with which someone 'diseased' has interacted, even if all rational knowledge points towards safety. Academics researching this have found that one third of the people they studied 'would not wear a laundered sweater previously worn by a person living with HIV/AIDS, nor would they drink out of a washed, sterilised glass that had been used a few days earlier by such a person'.[16] This extended beyond diseases we might think of as infectious: 'Contagion concerns could also be inferred from the tendency to avoid shaking hands with, or use silverware previously used by, people who have cancer.' Even though we know logically that these interactions can't infect us, our brains try to protect us from potential contamination. This affects how we might behave towards sick or impaired people, and also to the objects around them. I'm arguing that it changes how we behave towards the people standing beside them, too.

Stigma and the fallacy of choice

In the ancient empires of the world, such as the Greek and the Roman, foreign prisoners and slaves were tattooed to mark their criminality or their ownership, respectively. Indeed, it was so common that from the sixth century BCE onwards, slaves in ancient Greece were frequently referred to as 'stigmatici', or tattooed. Plato was a fan of this practice, writing in *The Laws*: 'If anyone is caught committing sacrilege, if he be a slave or a stranger, let his offence be written on his face and his hands.' And indeed, they did literally *write* the offence – records of commonly used stigmas include 'thief', and 'stop me, I'm a runaway' for slaves.[17] Today, we tend to use the word 'stigma' to mean the process and experience of being outcast or maligned in some way, due to a real or perceived characteristic. If you're stigmatised, the people around you experience you as deviating from their norms and comfort zones. People with physical impairments and mental illnesses are frequently stigmatised. This can be seen interpersonally, as we've explored, through practices like social rejection and exclusion, but also structurally, through the failure to organise our workplaces, communities, transport systems and so on in ways that can accommodate their needs. There are wonderful, brave campaigns to change this, but our interest here isn't in those who need care, but in those who provide it. Once again, we are harmed but overlooked.

Caregivers experience stigma both directly and indirectly. When our loved one is stigmatised, our lives are made harder indirectly. We carry the sorrow of watching that person be excluded, judged, and jeered at. For those caring for autistic people, evidence finds 'the impact of autism-related stigma upon caregiver mental health to be significant, meaningful and complex'.[18] Caregivers are also stigmatised directly. This is stigma by association, or what social scientists call 'associative stigma' (or alternatively, 'courtesy stigma'). Its impact on kin caregivers has barely been researched and, when it has, the focus has been on psychiatric situations. Based on my own experience and that of other caregivers, however, it's a widespread problem.

The extent to which we judge people, on any topic, depends on how much we think they should be able to control their own situation. So, for example, a blind person might be seen as more acceptable than an obese person, because we hold a cultural belief that obesity is controllable and a question of will power. Is caregiving controllable? Plainly not (unless we're sociopaths who don't care *about* each other and can therefore forgo caring *for* each other). However, my experience and that of the other caregivers and related experts with whom I've spoken suggests that our cultural belief is that it *should* be controllable. 'It's culturally expected that at some point, you put your parents into a home,' Karen told me. 'People ask me, "Are they going to transition [into a home]?", but I say only when they absolutely have to.'

Dr Camille Allard has studied caregivers, looking specifically at workplace policies that allow them to have special time off for their additional responsibilities, something we'll explore in Chapter 7. Working caregivers whom she interviewed told her they'd been interrogated for trying to access leave from work for their responsibilities. 'I had participants, for example, telling me that they had to justify . . . why they were caring for their grandparents or their brother,' she recounts. 'And very often, their manager will tell them, "Can't you find someone else?" There is such ignorance about the complexity of care relationships.' Her experience, and Karen's, show people assume that care is optional.

I have my own permutation of this experience. I was never interrogated as to why I was caring for my mum, but I was repeatedly told by colleagues and managers that I needed to rest more, do less outside work and take better care of myself. Those three things were true, but they were also infeasible. I couldn't rest more because I was bouncing between work and care all the time. If I was sick and off work, I still had to provide care. If I had a relative covering care for me, I still had to work. If there was a lull in my mum's symptoms, I never knew when that lull would end, so I was constantly on high alert. I was so burned out that when I did have time off work, I just got ill. I was writing my first book during a small part of my mother's illness, and various essays and articles, and this was a point of contention. If I was so overwhelmed, overloaded, over-everything, shouldn't I cull such superfluities? That's like telling someone stuck in a dark hole with a single crack of light to block that light out. Watching my mother grow sick and face an early death had, as poet Mary Oliver puts it, been 'as urgent as a knife' in its effect on me. I developed a deep-seated and steely resolve to pursue the dream I'd held since I was a small child: to be a writer. The belief that I could make this dream into reality was a vital antidote to the suffering around me. As caregivers, we receive these messages from colleagues, friends, neighbours and relatives: that we could be doing something differently, that if they were in our situation, they would do it differently, and by implication, better. By virtue of being close to someone who's unwell or in some way impaired, then, we become something to be avoided and something to be judged. Just when we need to be held and supported.

This creates a negative feedback loop, because caregivers internalise that stigma and begin to pre-empt it by self-stigmatising. In one study, forty-five per cent of kin caregivers for people with schizophrenia (a term used in the study, though now considered stigmatised by many activists) in India felt uncomfortable disclosing their family member's condition to others.[19] Specifically, they were concerned that disclosing the condition would harm not only the patient's marital prospects, but also their own, and those of other family members too. The mother-in-law of one woman with schizophrenia feared that her daughter-in-law's condition would reflect badly on her family, saying she felt that other people shouldn't know about it 'because they will start saying that if she has a mental illness, then why did we bring her as our daughter-in-law?'

Different countries have differing degrees of social acceptance of mental illness, but even in those that pride themselves on a high degree of such acceptance, are we really sure people wouldn't think we should make a different choice? Consider someone knowingly marrying a person with a gene for a severe degenerative disease – can you be certain there'd be no social judgement of their decision? No suggestion further down the line that they shouldn't need government or family support to provide care because 'they knew what they were getting into'? Needing care, and giving it, are cast as pathological. If you haven't avoided it sufficiently, it's your fault. And yet, unlike many stigmatised characteristics, we will all experience caregiving. In his seminal book

On the Mind: Confronting a Convenient Stigma

Stigma: Notes on the Management of Spoiled Identity, acclaimed social scientist Erving Goffman shares the story of a man who found himself slipping through the looking-glass and becoming stigmatised after many years of living a 'normal' life. He describes his situation: 'When I smelled an odour on the bus or subway before [my] colostomy, I used to feel very annoyed. I'd think people were awful, that they didn't take a bath . . . to me it seemed that they were filthy, dirty. Of course, at the least opportunity I used to change my seat.'[20] He says that he now thinks people must feel that way about him. By pathologising and being disgusted by others, he has done the same to himself.

Pointing to evolutionary causes of human behaviour, as with disease avoidance, can be viewed as determinist. If that's the way we're wired, then that's just the way it is, right? But the clue is in the word: *evolution*. It means 'a gradual process of change and development'.[21] To locate the partial cause of something in our evolution is not to say that it's fixed; rather, it's to say that it exists because of a gradual process of change, and so it can change further still. Likewise, stigmas can be removed. Consider populations that have been stigmatised historically and are now less so. LGBTQ people still experience stigma, discrimination and violence, but in many countries, huge leaps forward in rights, protections and social understanding have occurred. Likewise, mental illness is now part of an open conversation in many societies, rather than something to provoke shame and ostracisation. Or consider HIV and the appalling discrimination against its sufferers in its early years. Today, of course, this continues in many places, but there's also much more understanding of how

175

HIV is contracted and how to be safe in proximity to people with it. There are so many examples of us evolving our social understandings of each other that we can afford to have a little hope.

Making change happen

We can't change anything until we accept first that caregivers are an overlooked category of people experiencing social stigmatisation and exclusion. I bet if I'd asked you before you read this chapter to list socially excluded groups of people, you wouldn't have mentioned caregivers. Once we've accepted that, we need to recognise that those absurd tips to 'keep the flame alive' and so on aren't good enough: we require collective interventions.

Consider our education, whether that's school-based curricula or the education we imbibe through public information campaigns or similar. Caregiving and death are nowhere to be seen. Why have they been left out in the cold? Like I said in Chapter 1, trying to explain to people what this book was about while writing it – no, it's not about paid care workers, no, it's not about care homes and the state of social care, and so on – demonstrated the invisibility of caregivers, despite them making up the majority of those who provide care today, in rich and poor countries alike. Slowly, my interlocutors would start to mention people they knew who were caregiving – a woman across the road, an aunt, a work colleague who always had to leave suddenly. It would be as if they'd put on a new pair of spectacles, a sudden realisation dawning that, all around them, people were struggling with this thing they had previously either not noticed or been keen not to notice.

This *noticing* is the first step towards a collective psyche that can welcome caregiving rather than fear and reject it. Noticing can be midwifed by education; we need to teach caregiving in school curricula alongside the other lessons that focus on the development of people into functioning human beings, like civics, home education, sexual health and financial education.

Not all caregiving is for people who are dying, but when it is, there are innovative attempts to cultivate more social comfort with death, which might improve things. At 'death cafés', people gather to discuss death. The US organisation The Dinner Party connects grieving adults aged twenty to forty-ish so that they can share and support each other. There are also 'death doulas', able to support the process of dying, like the more conventional birth doula. However, all of these are usually interacted with by people who are already bereaved or on its cusp. Proximity to death becomes an exclusive club, rather than just . . . life.

We've also seen that there's substantial work to be done addressing the stigmatisation and discrimination experienced by caregivers. Each of us may like to think that we are immune to bias, but just as we're unlikely to be the sole survivor of a plane crash or the lonely heroic escapee from a fire, nor are we devoid of bias. Much work has been done to expose the implicit prejudices we hold towards different categories of people, for example around women and competency in the workplace, or racialised people and laziness. It's time to recognise that caregivers are also on the receiving end of implicit bias, and to include them in endeavours to undo those harms. This could lead to better support and inclusion within social networks and at institutions like workplaces. As we've seen in the preceding pages, becoming a caregiver can be a huge shock to people, affecting their sense of time, identity and purpose. If we had all been taught that caregiving is natural and something to support and include instead of avoid and reject, that transition would be easier.

The risk with talking about things like disease avoidance and implicit bias is that we lose hope. If we're wired this way, maybe we're just doomed to stay exclusionary, stigmatising and biased? I do not think we can ever eradicate these elements of humanity. But we can develop better awareness of when they're being activated, and a stronger muscle to then choose whether we wish to follow their cues. With this in place, perhaps those friends of Karen's wouldn't imply she should be institutionalising her parents. Perhaps Dr Allard's interviewees wouldn't be interrogated by their employers, and maybe I wouldn't have faced consternation and judgement for my choices and seeming inability to get on top of life. Perhaps neighbours would be more likely to offer support, to do a weekly shop or simply sit with the person who needs care for an hour once a week. Perhaps it would be a world in which people are taught that caregiving is natural, and that if they encounter caregivers in their daily life, at work or in their communities or elsewhere, there's nothing to back away from, but rather something to lean toward.

*   *   *

After the breakup with that curly-haired green-eyed man, I wanted to die. I know now that I was suffering from deep depression and total burnout. But all I knew then was that I needed an end to everything, that sweet-sounding eternal oblivion. I planned how I'd do it. I wrote my passwords and pin codes out so that it would be easier to mop up my life after I'd gone. I examined diagrams of knots online and considered the ceiling fixtures most likely to hold my suspended weight. I set a date for its completion, when I thought my mum should be out of the woods after her transplant. Everything had gone dark.

I'm still here for several reasons. Partly, because I found an amazing psychotherapist who was so kind, so wise and so skilled. Friends stepped up, scooping me warmly into their homes and coping admirably with the brittle, maudlin mess before them. Medication helped too. And, of course, deep down, I suppose I always knew I couldn't leave my mum while she needed me. In a way, although caregiving had brought me to the edge, the responsibility that came with it also stopped me from going over. All those elements were vital. And so, too, was the undoing of my own denial of death. My mum's sickness, the constant proximity to suffering in hospital, the way that so many parts of myself seemed to be steeped in death and negativity . . . It was a moment of choice: give up or find a new way to exist with the facts of that existence. I realised that while much of my suffering couldn't be addressed by changes of perspective, such as the very physical need for rest, shifting how I understood what was happening could salve my mental suffering. I made friends with mortality. I understood that it simply 'is'. This ended the jarring dissonance of inhabiting a world that pretends otherwise, while every day being confronted with the opposite. I embraced the knowledge of our creatureliness, eking out fleeting private moments to lie with the notion that we are nothing but briefly colliding particles.

Who Cares

'Come to terms with death,' said Albert Camus, the French existentialist philosopher. 'Thereafter, anything is possible.'[22]

Perhaps it seems like a tall order. I'm saying that to address the caregiver's mind, we need to start by changing ourselves and our collective psychology. But haven't we done that before, many times over, and on many things? Human societies have believed in gods inside natural objects, in gods in the sky, in a god that created everything in the world, and in no god at all. Before Freud, the idea that adult neuroses might be due to childhood experiences would have seemed totally bizarre. Now, it's hard to understand them differently. The idea that all humans should be considered to have inalienable rights did not exist before we made it so. Like our bodies, our psyches evolve. But unlike our bodies, if we want to direct that psychological evolution towards specific ends, we must take conscious, intentional steps towards them before we're sure they'll come into being. Let's teach our children that we're creatures, just like every other living thing. Let's teach them to learn to respond, rather than react, to stimuli. Let's teach them that to care for one another, especially when someone is in need, is a beautiful thing: a thing possibly more important than anything else in our world.

CHAPTER 6

On Freedom: The Lie of the Individual

'Do you sometimes want to wake up to the
singularity
we once were?
  – Marie Howe, excerpt from 'Singularity'

'I have this weird thing that if I sleep with someone, they're going to take my creativity through my vagina.' So said pop artist and avant-garde fashion icon Lady Gaga in a 2010 interview with *Vanity Fair*.[1] Around sixty years before this somewhat startling confession, Simone de Beauvoir had described a similar concern in rather more erudite language. In her seminal feminist text, *The Second Sex*, the French philosopher expounded on the condition of woman. Woman, Beauvoir wrote, was relegated to the daily drudgery of domestic labour, in contrast to man who can embark on projects that create things above and beyond the mundane: '. . . she is condemned to domestic labour, which locks her into repetition . . . day after day it repeats itself in identical form from century to century; it produces nothing new. Man's case is radically different. He does not provide for the group in the way worker bees do, by a simple vital process, but rather by acts that transcend his animal condition.'[2] The role accorded to women by society is deemed, by Gaga and Beauvoir, to take from us our creative potential, the many projects we might engender if we weren't so busy with the mundane. Their sentiment is one I used to hold myself, and is no doubt part of the reason why I struggled with my sudden role of caregiver.

In the previous chapter, we explored the psychological hardship of care: the burnout, depression, compassion fatigue and overwhelm that many experience. I certainly felt I was living in a long, dark tunnel much of the time that my mum was sick, one I was simultaneously desperate to escape and terrified of leaving in case the only exit was by her dying. I think care is always hard, but made much harder when it contradicts what we've been told to expect from life. I'd been taught to expect what I presume many men have always expected – a right to choose my path in life. When I encountered people living in more gendered patterns, it angered me, and I had a righteous sense that they were living incorrectly. In Chapter 2, I recounted my rage at discovering that the middle-aged men I met hiking alone on the Coast to Coast trail were leaving their wives to care for their own mothers back home, their domestic division apparently not one of labour, but one of labour for the woman and exhilaration for the man. Where was the women's freedom? Didn't they understand that women could now be independent, autonomous selves, just as men had long been? My rage was both legitimate and flawed. It was legitimate because the gender split between free and not-free was so apparent. Here were men, once again freeloading on women's caregiving. However, it was flawed because focusing on the gender asymmetry blinded me to the deeper problem: that the idol of the independent, free self, unbound by mundane domesticity and able to go on long-distance hikes without a second glance, is a false one. None of us are free in the way that matters from a caregiving perspective, nor should we wish to be. To pay witness to caregivers, we need to understand this, interrogating the foundations of false independence on which we've built our societies.

Civil liberties are those freedoms that are protected in law and against which governments should not impinge. They're enshrined in the US Bill of Rights, and in human rights acts and conventions; they're embodied in the Statue of Liberty, and articulated in the declarations of revolutions from India to France. Freedom in this sense aims to protect us from arbitrary rulers, from colonisers and mad kings. Unfortunately – and perhaps because most historical political writing was performed by men, who were not the primary caregivers of humanity – this application of freedom didn't stop at government. The great men of history – and some of the present, too – have constructed an ideal-typical person who is independent instead of dependent, self-sufficient instead of needy, rational instead of emotion-driven. He is certainly not someone who needs, or is obliged to give, care. At most, he may oversee it, taking masterly responsibility for its delegation, but he doesn't deliver such a repetitious and animalistic requirement himself. You won't catch him bed-bathing loved ones or standing dazed in supermarket aisles, trying to figure out which food might tempt someone whose tastebuds have been twisted by chemo. Liberty has been valorised and being dependent on others has been pathologised. Professor Joan Tronto has written that 'rather than viewing dependency as a natural part of the human experience, political theorists emphasise dependence as the character-destroying condition'.[3] Dependency is something that's feared, that entails belittlement and infantilisation. The 'right' way to be is free, and so we seek to offload the duties of our furtive dependencies, either to an underclass of slaves, to women in the home, to migrant women workers, or, as we explored in Chapter 3, to machines. The ideal person instead can spend their time in pursuit of greatness or pleasure. In his 1891 essay, 'The Soul of Man Under Socialism', Oscar Wilde wrote: 'It is mentally and morally injurious to man to do anything in which he does not find pleasure . . . Man is made for something better than disturbing dirt.' He asserted: 'All unintellectual labour, all monotonous, dull labour, all labour that deals with dreadful things, and involves unpleasant conditions, must be done by machinery.' Wilde is railing at the conditions of the labourer forced to do tedious activities because he needs his wage to survive, but simultaneously, he inveighs against doing anything that involves monotony or 'unpleasant conditions'. I wonder how Wilde would have reacted to a loved one needing care, certainly a monotonous and unpleasant job at times.

We can see a similar sentiment at an international level, taking the case of the United Nations and how it writes about caregiving. Time-use surveys are its recommended tool to expose how care is apportioned within the household. These surveys quantify how much time is spent doing specific tasks, such as caregiving, and so provide evidence of the unseen and unpaid labour that keeps our world going. In turn, the UN reports, 'policies that take into account the care and domestic functions at home are better poised to release households from time-burdens and make them available for leisure or economic activities'.[4] The assumption is that it would be good to quantify caregiving time in order to liberate us for leisure or paid work. In Wilde's case, care is something to be ignored – something we don't have to do. In the UN's case, care is something we should make visible, but only in order to reduce it, jettisoning it in favour of better pursuits, which are, apparently, 'leisure or paid work'.

But we are not free. We never have been, we never will be and never can be. It is not our nature. When we inculcate the idea that human beings can be free – can avoid doing things they don't wish to, can control their own destinies, and have a right to that control – we set ourselves up for enormous personal pain when caregiving comes knocking. It shocks us when our destiny is suddenly shaped by forces beyond our control or imagination. And it makes the literal tasks of caregiving more difficult, because when a culture only respects those without needs, it makes it shameful to be someone with them. This makes our caregiving lives much harder, because those who need support with daily living can be angry, frustrated and ashamed by their condition and their apparent failure to live up to this fictional ideal of the free individual. We've heard already from several caregivers, including myself, that those for whom we've cared have rejected outside help even when it was sorely needed by us, to protect our physical and mental health from ruin.

And within the direct caring relationship itself, too, the ideal of being an active, independent individual causes problems. At the start of 2018, my mum became extremely unwell. She didn't explain quite how unwell, and so it was only when she was close to death that she called for help. She'd had a massive allergic reaction to some of her cancer medication. There she was, hooked up and bleeping in intensive care, her heart under so much pressure it developed an arrhythmia. She apologised for not alerting me sooner because she 'hadn't wanted to bother anyone'. It was one of many incidents when I had to read her the riot act and demand different behaviour in future, a main ingredient in the slow reversal of our mother-daughter identities.

In the previous chapter, I recounted that one of the most common responses when people learned I was caring for my mother was 'I couldn't do that' or some permutation on that theme. The way we live now, and the underlying beliefs we hold, mean that nobody wants to countenance that such a cruel and unexpected thing could collide with their lives. Don't misunderstand me; I held those beliefs too. I absolutely hated losing my freedom to care. I craved desperately a weekend when I could do exactly as I pleased, when I could know for certain that I wouldn't suddenly be at a hospital. But it was a category error, because I had never truly been free to begin with. I just didn't realise it.

The billiard ball fallacy

One night during her illness, I dreamed about my mum and me. In fact, I dreamed about her often, but usually these dreams were nightmares: her face screaming, her body drawn backwards into darkness, a formless beast coming at me that I suddenly knew was her . . . But this dream was different. I'm not sure whether it was good or bad; like much of care, the lines between the two are blurred. I dreamed that her veins were places of darkness, black highways through her tired limbs. Lights appeared in them, dancing like car headlamps at night but less uniform and many-coloured. They fizzed and danced through the black spaces under her skin, which I wished achingly I could reach into and clean out. Then I saw my own arm outstretched, my own veins turning black, too, the boundary between me and her dissolving, if it was ever there in the first place. And then the lights were coruscating in my veins just like hers, so pretty and so deadly, spreading their bright violence through us both.

When I woke, I wondered if it was a premonition: I was so tired, so broken by it all, that it didn't seem a stretch to believe I might also have cancer. Wouldn't that be something, I thought, both of us rigged up to all those bleepers, with a plastic tube through the crook of my arm into somewhere near my heart, just like hers? We could lie in twin beds in a shared room. We could grumble quietly about the quality of the tea – not that we'd be able to keep it down. I could look over and see her hand, puffy and freckled. We could smile our moonchild skulls at each other and begin to dance with the lights, making a joined river of our cancers to drown in together.

That dream was a depiction of how deeply linked I felt to my mother throughout her sickness and dying. The only word I can find to capture the visceral sensation is 'umbilically': just as I'd been tethered to her at my own entry into the world, so she seemed to be tethered to me in her exit. Sometimes this made me angry. I hadn't chosen to have children yet, and here I was, mothering my mother with all the enormous love and pain of parenthood. Sometimes it left me in awe of how deeply entwined we can feel to one another. Mostly, it made me acutely aware that I had never been free in the first place; I'd only been in waiting for this time when my dormant unfreedom would wake.

Our unfreedom is not a case of opinion, even if for you, unlike me, it hasn't yet made itself the main theme of your life. We are factually unfree and factually interdependent. This is the case at every level of existence, and it's an indictment of our world that it takes something like a serious illness or accident to make us wake up to it. Our climate crisis is teaching us that we're interdependent at a global level. Even the body and brain turn out to be biologically interdependent with those of others. Historically, much neuroscience was conducted as if the human brain stood alone in the world, with scientists observing individual brains without consideration of interaction and whether it might alter what was being seen. Now, neuroscientists are exploring 'brain-to-brain coupling' in their work: the idea that the system of one brain can be coupled to another, and that this coupling affects what we think and do. It seems that we don't think *for ourselves* but *with others*. Our wider bodies, too, are linked to one another's at a deeply animal level. Scientists have proven that social support reduces stress and brings a range of physical health benefits. Conversely, social isolation is bad for our health. Perhaps most surprisingly, they've also discovered that social rejection can literally cause us pain, just like breaking your arm. Social connection isn't just something we like to have, but instead something that shapes how we live at a biological level as well as a social one. We didn't know these biological facts historically. Perhaps for that reason, and because much of our scholarship was performed by those with the least need to consider dependency, i.e. men, our notion of the self (in the white Western world) has also been misinformed.

Psychologist Hope Landrine explored this interconnectedness in her lifetime, questioning the idea of our 'selves' that we hold, just as I had to question mine as my umbilical tethering to my mother became apparent. Landrine wrote: 'While assumptions about what a self is are furthest from our conscious awareness, they also are the most powerful and significant assumptions behind and beneath our behaviour.'[5] And just as your assumptions about what you are will shape whether you want a family, or what kind of work you do, they also shape how you'll approach caregiving, and whether you'll expect it before it comes for you. Landrine explains that in the individualistic idea of the self, 'the self is represented as existing free of any and all contexts: the self is here; the context is there . . . [this self] can be described without reference to others or to a context'.[6] This independent self, separate to everything around it, interacts with others in the way that billiard balls interact – separate, hard-shelled spheres bumping into each other. That bump may, at most, shift their trajectory, but it will not leave them fundamentally altered. Alternatively, we can conceive of the self as *part of* everything around it, rather than as *separate from*. That version of the self 'is created and recreated in interactions and contexts, and exists only in and through these'. In the billiard ball version of the self, it would be strange to be dependent on other people, or for our personalities, choices and so on to be shaped by them too deeply. It makes no sense because we're hard-shelled, separate spheres. Anyone who was dependent on others, then, would be wrong in some way. They'd be pathologised and, by proxy, so would those caring for them. Sound familiar? Only the parent–child relationship is given a hall pass, until an age at which maturity is assumed. This has real, practical impacts on the daily lives of caregivers. We saw in Chapter 5 how caregivers are interrogated by employers as if we should all be free of dependents. The very existence of the carebots we met in Chapter 3 is partly because we believe we shouldn't be providing care ourselves. The atomised conventional family, on its lonely island, and the weird novelty of 'kinning', is also a product of this false idea of the self.

When I came across American philosopher Martha Nussbaum's assertion that we are 'both capable and needy', I knew I'd found a perfect encapsulation of what caregiving teaches about 'our-selves'.[7] We've forgotten that we're not just beings with projects and pursuits, but also beings that love and have needs. When Nussbaum describes us as needy, what does this word conjure up for you? The example sentence for needy provided by an online dictionary is this: 'As he became more competent and less needy, his interpersonal relationships improved.' Neediness, then, is commensurate with incompetence. For our lives to be better, we should be less needy. It is assuredly not a desirable condition. Yet take stock, for a moment, of your needs. You are needy as hell. You need money, so you need a job. You need shelter and food with some nutritional value. You need human interaction, ideally not through a screen, as we saw in Chapter 3. Sometimes, you probably need someone to bring you soup or aspirin because you're sick. You need doctors. Maybe right now you can walk and go to the toilet alone, but you couldn't always, and probably won't be able to in the future. Our human condition is one of neediness. Capitalism tends to obscure this in its construction of the 'free worker' – a person contracted for a job and paid in return is not a slave, so he is free. But of course, though he may not be a slave, he is still needy. He is, actually, a dependent of his employer, and his employer, too, is dependent on workers coming to work, doing their jobs and fuelling the engine of profit. Without each other, they'll be dependents of the government or of charity.

Rehabilitation of the ideas of neediness and dependency away from infantilising connotations of childhood and disparaging assumptions of incompetence is vital for addressing our care crisis. If we need to move away from those ideas, what do we move towards? What's the alternative to the billiard ball? The answer comes to us from feminist scholarship – perhaps unsurprisingly, given how the responsibility for caregiving is allotted in our world. Autonomy means self-government. It comes from the Greek *autos* ('self') and *nomos* ('custom, law'). Being autonomous means being able and allowed to act upon motives and values that we recognise as our own. It's important because it allows us to make decisions for ourselves, such as whether we wish to prioritise work or care, whether we want to be cared for by machines or humans, and so on. Respecting another person's autonomy means not trying to coerce them or override their wishes. However, it's often assumed to mean a person can act, feel and exist entirely alone, as if they're the only human in the world, and that to act from that position is in fact rational and good. But if we understand that we're not billiard balls at all, but, like my dream about my veins and my mum's joining themselves like two rivers meeting, deeply interconnected to each other, inextricable from brain to body to soul, then it follows that our autonomy can only exist within those relations too.

Feminist theorists have termed this notion 'relational autonomy'; our sense of self arises out of our relations. We know ourselves through and because of our relationships with parents, teachers, friends, lovers and so on. And when we make choices for ourselves, we're able to make them because of that web of relationships. Good caregiving is the epitome of this interweaving of autonomy and relationships. Caregiving, when it's done well, doesn't seek to do everything for the recipient, but rather to do what the recipient can't and to enable what they can. This is why Ulla calls herself her husband's 'possibility maker', a term that felt like a sky clearing of clouds when she told me it, so clearly did it describe the more joyful, hopeful aspect of being a caregiver.

I certainly saw myself, at times, as the enabler of my mother's autonomy. In her final months in summer 2020, she could no longer walk more than a few steps, but she didn't want a wheelchair. Her general approach to being sick was to be angry and refuse the things that might mitigate some of her losses. She was loath to accept her new status as needy, repetitively suggesting that tomorrow might be 'a better day', though of course that tomorrow never came. Eventually, after I'd found a company from which we could rent a lightweight, foldable wheelchair that she had to admit was good value and wouldn't take up too much space, and I'd pointed out equally repetitively that she loved being out on the river path, and that I'd love to take her out on it, but we needed a wheelchair to do so, she accepted it and we ordered the contraption. It was a clever design, folding like a concertina to a third of its size, and light enough to carry down the stairs outside her front door without strain. Once we had it, she was thrilled to be back outside, as I'd known she would be. Sometimes, after I'd wheeled her close enough to the river wall, she'd even manage a few steps on her own out of the chair. One of my final photos of her is from the last time we did this: her standing there, her hands on the wall, wearing a dark, padded coat with a fur-trimmed hood, her face turned away from the camera as she looks out on the river and the city behind it, drinking in the view she loved so much. I went back a year later and took the same photo without her standing in it, an attempt to accept and observe her absence. And now that she's gone, and my own autonomy is unconstrained in many ways compared to when she was alive, I'm still deeply bound up with her, to our ways of relating to each other, to the experiences we shared and battled. No person who's been a caregiver could sensibly think that we stand as single, independent individuals.

*　　　*　　　*

Who Cares

Of course, you may be reading this as someone who has no dependants. It may seem that I'm talking about something either so abstract as to be irrelevant to you, or so specific as to be too removed from your own experience. Consider, then, this more familiar idea as an analogy. Many of us will be familiar with the notion that we're all closer to destitution than we like to think. For example, in June 2021, it was reported that fifty-nine per cent of Americans are only one pay cheque away from homelessness.[8] The UK fares similarly. We need to have the same notion for caregiving. Anyone in our lives, at any time, can need care, through sickness, accident or old age. Car crashes happen. Cancers happen. Mental health crises happen. It doesn't matter whether you have children or not, a spouse or not; if you love *anyone*, and you're not an asshole, the need to care is waiting in the wings. If you are 'free' for now, consider how many flukes and fortunes upon which that freedom rests. 'Freedom' is always contingent. Our failure to recognise this is why caregiving hits people's lives like a bus. It's also why so many people lack care today, and why so many of our laws and policies fail to enable us to provide care.

After Carlyle Brown's wife Barbara had a stroke, he wrote a play about their experience, called 'A Play by Barb & Carl'. In it, a character explains:

> You see, the reason we have [medical] insurance is because the world is a dangerous place. Anything can happen . . . Anything. Anything, anytime, anywhere, stuff happens. And to be sick, in poor health where you are being betrayed by your own body . . .

the most unkind cut of them all . . . stuff happens. And the question is not whether, but when it will happen to you. Because we know it will happen to you. We just don't know when. So, we have to protect ourselves. We have to protect ourselves from every eventuality whatsoever. We need insurance to assure ourselves that come those rainy days, in the end, everything is going to be okay. The trouble is that type of vigilance is expensive. Luck is for free, but it doesn't come with any guarantees. Whatever it is, you're going to have to pay. They got you by the scalpel. I mean, they just can't give it away. And sometimes all you can do is pay your premium and pray you don't get sick. Because, you see, you never know when you might need somebody to bring you a glass of water . . . to raise you up . . . to lend you a hand . . .

When you can't afford insurance, then the insurance you need is your family, your loved ones, the kindness of strangers. You need somebody. And Lord help you if you haven't paid your premium on that . . . paid your premium on love.

Carlyle and Barb, like me, fell through the looking-glass, from the world in which people believe they can 'stand on their own two feet' to the world in which they are interdependent and, as Nussbaum said, both capable and needy. Our neediness means we will, at some point, require a community around us that can become our care network. When that community is too small, or indeed just one person, it puts enormous strain on the caregiver and creates feelings of guilt in the recipient. So, we must pay our premium on love, because that love will cushion us when we are bruised. We need that wider notion of family, that kinning practice, to survive these situations. And that starts from recognising that we're not free individuals, but intertwined beings who need each other, always.

Even in countries with robust and broad government provision of care, this will remain the case. This is partly due to the nature of government and partly due to the nature of care. Government provision of services is often taken to be synonymous with equal provision of services, i.e. if we have a good government owning and running our services, then everyone will get the assistance they need and it'll be fairly distributed. That's not what happens. Whether services are provided by the private sector or by governments, or some sort of deal between them, 'postcode lotteries' always exist. Line knows that many people from other countries think life is comparatively easy in her native Norway. She was at pains in our interview to make clear that that's not always the case. Although her son has great free provision, such as day care and respite care, she told me that this is partly because she lives in Skien, a city. If she was in a more rural area, there'd be fewer services available. Her son can get free housing now that he's over eighteen, and they've applied for it, but they might wait years because housing stock is limited.

In summer 2020, my mother's cancer returned after her remission. She was told it was terminal, but – that wonderful three-letter word that beckoned our hearts – *but,* there was a wonder drug called lenalidomide that couldn't cure her, but might prolong her life. Her consultant oncologist had to write to a board to get it approved for her, because the cost was so high, at around £10,000 for a month's supply. We held the box carefully, passing it between us like curators handling a priceless antique. She very much wanted the additional weeks or months alive that it could bring. It made her incredibly sick. Her steroids were increased and a new anti-nausea medicine was prescribed, one that came in the same sort of packaging in which you get perfume samples in women's magazines – a pastel-coloured cardboard cover, a single pill surrounded by empty pastel space. None of it worked, and the lenalidomide made her too unwell to continue. Her quality of life wasn't worth it for what little extra time it would give. She was able to get the drug because she was relatively young for someone dying, and because her oncologist was highly thought of and at a very respected hospital in London. But many don't meet this criteria, and decisions by the UK's National Health Service not to approve cancer drugs because of the expense make regular scandalous headlines. In Scandinavia, my interviewees were at pains to tell me that everything is not the same for everyone, despite publicly funded services. Lotteries exist in both government-run and private-sector services; swapping one for the other merely moves the location of blame, not the problem.

The COVID-19 possibility

It's all well and good to say we need to pay our premium on love, to nurture relationships and become expert at kinning, but these are just words. How do we do it practically? COVID-19 can help. By April 2020, more than half of the world's population was under lockdown orders as the COVID-19 virus spread around the globe.[9] For those with underlying health conditions or impaired immune systems, venturing out at all, even to buy basic provisions, was too dangerous. And even if you were lucky enough to be in good health, if you'd been in contact with someone who tested positive, you were under a stay-at-home order. Life became acutely bipolar: we kept our eyes glued to the rolling news updates –Wuhan, Italy, London – while simultaneously turning our attention to our neighbourhoods – did we know anyone nearby? If we had to stay at home, who would fetch the things we needed? In the UK, panic-buying of over-the-counter pain relief medication saw paracetamol's price jump by up to thirty per cent.[10] A seller from Sri Lanka listed 240 tablets for £12,500 on eBay.[11] Did you know someone locally who might slip you a tablet if you were in desperate need?

My mother's symptoms seemed to be easing at that time. However, as a severely immunocompromised person, she had to stay in her house to stay alive. Even things delivered to her were dangerous, swarming as they might be with COVID-19 germs. She was gutted. It was the first time in a couple of years that she could have carefully begun going out and about in a more normal way. She'd still have needed to avoid public transport because of her poor immunity, but going to a café, a local gallery or the supermarket were possible once again. And then they weren't – for any of us. For Christmas, mere months before, I'd bought her a keyring saying 'Strong, capable and brave' to encourage her back into the world and to health. Lockdown meant it lay forlornly on the table, gathering dust. We were all bereft of those simple, taken-for-granted pleasures, but she most of all, because they'd been her light at the end of the tunnel. We didn't know then, of course, that in a few months' time the cancer would return, and she'd be dead a handful more after that. For the first few weeks of the pandemic, I didn't go to see her. I was laid up sick, the virus that had been plaguing me for months rearing its head again, and we were also worried by the idea I might transmit COVID-19 to her. So the question was this: if she couldn't go to the shops, and I couldn't visit her, how would she get food? The supermarket delivery services were entirely booked up for many weeks ahead with people panic-buying. She knew some of her neighbours, but in the way that so many of us 'know' our neighbours today – they were acquainted, they might comment on the weather or the state of the shared refuse store in passing, but little more. My mother was very 'English' – asking for help was far from easy – perhaps less easy than starving.

It was, then, an enormous relief when a local group was created to provide community support in her area. It was one of many established across the country, and across the world, in response to the pandemic. In the USA, Liam Elkind became one of the stars of the show. A junior at Yale University, Elkind described watching the pandemic and feeling powerless, especially when he thought of the frontline workers, like his father, who was a doctor. A friend, Simone Policano, posted on Facebook asking if anyone knew how to connect young volunteers with older and immunocompromised people, and Elkind suggested they start a service that did just that. Invisible Hands was born: essentially a sort of Amazon Prime for the vulnerable, with no delivery charges.[12] Its service has been much-needed, but for all its good, I believe it's fatally flawed. If we consider the distribution of power and abilities within such a model, it's evident that it follows a classic charity approach – the better-offs provide for the worse-offs. We're categorised into more able or less able, independent or dependent. We all know which category we'd rather be in. We're blowing a kiss to relational autonomy, flirting with it while the well-meaning independent volunteers stay within their billiard-ball concept of selfhood. This can't undo the exclusion and stigmatisation of caregivers, nor teach us to kin as equals. We have to embed care in our communities, but if we do it in a way that entrenches these dichotomies, we'll win the battle at expense of the war. We need an alternative vision, underpinned by different beliefs.

Radical, concrete practice

We've already met the women of OWCH in their leafy north London abode. As we saw, they're part of a movement around the world that's trying to do things differently. Bruno Friedel is an expert on co-housing based at the University of Oxford. Serendipitously, he also happens to be the partner of a close friend who, when I mention that I think co-housing is part of the solution to the care crisis, connects me with him. I enjoy our conversation, my lonely passion for the topic reflected at me and enhanced with his expertise.

For Friedel, co-housing is about more than a segue from the traditional family to a chosen family, as we explored in Chapter 4. It can get to the very meat of the issue with which we're grappling here – our inescapable interdependence. It changes our concept of space, he tells me, shifting us from 'seeing co-housing as a limitation of the private household space to an expansion of the shared space . . . this makes us recognise that there are benefits of shared space and facilities, and that positive, organic forms of community can arise, whether that be from shared gardens, laundries, kitchens, or tool sheds.' He wasn't surprised at all when he heard I was interested in writing about co-housing in relation to care. 'It makes a whole lot of sense. It's a model that allows people to draw on their own networks, but also to create ones that are mutually supportive, while still gaining from the regular health and social care system. It's a model that makes a lot of intuitive sense, and recognises our interdependency in a way that's part of the fabric of our everyday lives.' He believes that co-housing can catalyse broader community care, too, with residents taking their ethic of interconnection into the surrounding neighbourhood. The women of OWCH echoed this sentiment, telling me: 'We're not a coven, we're not a clique, we're not a convent . . . we're part of the wider community.'

Co-housing is a deft strategy for paying your premium on love. Crucially, it doesn't presume to divide people into 'useful' versus 'needy'. People's different skills, abilities and temperaments mean they contribute what makes sense for them; everyone is different but equal. The gifts of support that occur within co-housing exemplify the way in which care is a big life drama made up of thousands of smaller acts – collection from a hospital appointment, grocery shopping done for you, a meal cooked, an understanding face listening to dilemmas about medication. It's not the specialist, hands-on care that severe impairments require, and on which we'll touch in Chapter 8, but it's the bulk of caring that takes place today in a world with high rates of chronic illness and lengthy, frail old ages. Of course, we may not wish, or be able, to live in co-housing. That's where Hilary Cottam comes in.

Cottam is an award-winning social innovator based in the UK. Her career is illustrious and cosmopolitan. In the late 1980s, she supported famine-relief work in northern Ethiopia, later moving to live in the barrio of La Ciénaga in the Dominican Republic and working on a range of community projects. Over the past twenty-odd years, she's been troubleshooting the design of social institutions such as schools, prisons and care services, mainly in the UK. When I hear a term like 'social innovator', I'm often tempted to roll my eyes. What does it actually *mean*? What are they actually *doing*? Are they going to try to tell me their new app will solve everything? But Cottam's work is compelling, bringing fresh ways of thinking about problems together with what she terms 'radical, concrete practice'. In her lucid and urgent book, *Radical Help: How We Can Remake the Relationships Between Us and Revolutionise the Welfare State*, Cottam took on the care crisis, along with other salient issues of our time. The UK welfare state is evidently unable to cope with the escalating need of those with disabilities or impairments. With a rare and beautiful fearlessness, Cottam and her team were determined not to be bound by path dependencies and conventional approaches, and elected instead to observe the issues, listen to the people experiencing them and build, brick by brick, from there, until something new and effective appeared.

In the case of caregiving, they designed something called Circle, which is 'part social club, part concierge service, and part cooperative self-help group'. It aimed to be 'a system that made the most of the horizontal bonds, enabling older people to support and connect with each other'. She and her team secured a start-up grant from local government and set up two telephone lines. They bought some gardening and DIY tools, and asked local people if they'd like to join this new thing. They could call the free phone number at any time for practical support, or to relay an idea for a new activity they'd like to arrange. There was a membership fee of £30 per person, an aspect that other comparable initiatives, like the Village model in some US neighbourhoods, have replicated, often with a sliding scale according to income. This has provoked concerns – is this a form of privatisation? Shouldn't government be providing these kinds of services for free? When we spoke, Cottam explained that Circles are initially started with local government funding, and that members have 'pushed back hard' against criticisms of the use of fees. 'It was quite interesting to see,' she tells me, recounting a specific incident in which a journalist interviewing Circle members asked about this aspect. 'The members' concept was, we have an organisation that we own and we run; it's ours. We decide. We don't have to go to some board to ask them to provide balloon classes or trampolining classes or whatever. We're in control, and we're helping each other. Why would we want the local government to organise that for us?'

The sentiment Cottam describes is allied with those held by the women of OWCH, who hold fast to self-determination as a collective – or 'we shall not be done unto', as Maria Brenton puts it.

Circle worked, and astonishingly well. The phone lines were very busy – members called for help with everything from cinema trips to sick pets and dripping taps. The four staff members were there to find solutions or simply provide reassurance. Members suggested the activities they'd like to do, working together through Circle to bring them to life. Nobody is 'befriended'; rather, they exercise their autonomy within a web of relationships and the choices created by being part of that web. The facilitating staff members keep track of everything using a digital platform known as a Customer Relationship Management (CRM) system: 'This simple piece of technology changed the boundaries of what was possible. Each Circle, with a small team of four, could keep track of a membership of over one thousand (with a potential capacity for double that number), understanding what each member might like and need, reminding us when the anniversary of a loved one's death might come around or when help was needed with that crucial hospital check-up.' In the US, the aforementioned Village Movement is somewhat comparable: older people come together in a locale to provide self-governed mutual support.[13] These models are the sibling of co-housing, creating connection across a broader geographical spread and bringing interdependency into the light in creative and effective ways.

The real test of Circle was whether it could create stronger bonds between its members, rather than merely give its staff plenty to do at their behest. Cottam recounts the story of Belinda, who'd been a member of Circle for some time when she notified the staff that she was going into hospital for a knee operation. One of them called her to find out what support she'd need upon her discharge.

'Oh no,' Belinda responded, 'Florence is doing the shopping, Tony is doing the garden, and Melissa and Jo are popping in to cook and chat.'

Circle was alive and breathing on its own. It's effective for many reasons, including that it neutralises some of the stigma around neediness. Firstly, there are many members, so rather than asking only one person to help with something, you're putting your need to a whole body of people, and those with the time and energy will step forward. This reduces the feeling that you're a burden. And because Circle isn't static – it doesn't offer a small selection of fixed activities, but instead is continually designed and redesigned by the members' ideas and abilities – members will experience themselves as both givers and takers.

When Cottam met him, Stan was eighty-nine years old and largely housebound and isolated. He sat alone each day, yearning to be able to hear music in the company of others as he used to love doing. Together, they created a telephone music club, just in time for Stan's ninetieth birthday, and for him to experience the joy of six people on the line, wishing him a happy birthday and enjoying the music with him. Stan couldn't do much physically, but he could be part of something, contributing with music selection and conversation, being an equal but different part of the whole, like everyone else. Because Circle is organised by humans, for humans, rather than being some production-line concept of care and need, someone like Stan, who has given the joy of the music club to its attendees, will know that next time he needs taking to a doctor's appointment in someone's car, it's part of a reciprocal exchange.

Secondly, you are in an environment in which periodic

neediness and dependency are normalised. This week, Belinda needs support. Perhaps next week, Tony will. And so on. This would have worked well for my mum. The idea that she was the sick one, incapable and incapacitated, was deeply uncomfortable for her. She needed ways for the world to see that she still had value. She was part of a book group with women in her local area, and had loved it before she got sick. During lockdown, with everyone unable to leave home, it became possible for her to participate again, because her own incapacity was mimicked in everyone else's. I taught her to use Zoom, and suddenly she was emailing them all and running their meetings online. She felt like herself again, just a little. It took a global pandemic for that little bit of dignity to be restored to her, that small crumb of participation. With Circle, it could have been different.

Organisations like OWCH and Circle have at their heart a horizontal, rather than vertical, idea of power. Relationships are webs, not one-way streets. Before the welfare state and the government provided income replacement for unemployment or those unable to work due to an accident or sickness, a version of this was common in the form of 'friendly societies'. These were groups of people who paid an equal amount into a shared pot. In return, if they hit hard times, a payment could be made to them. Then, governments (not all, but many) took over responsibility for financially supporting citizens who experienced accidents or illness and couldn't work as a result, and friendly societies died out. Those societies were focused, largely, on money: collecting it to redistribute it when the need arose. Some friendly societies included other elements, like social gatherings or care visits (though the latter were also sometimes inspections in case the sick person was pretending to avoid work!), but the primary function was financial insurance. Today, we need more than financial insurance. We need that love premium.

Etymologically, the word 'innovate' comes from the Latin *innovare*, meaning 'to renew' or 'to restore'. It's a signal to us that, rather than trying to conjure up something 'new', we would do better to restore and remember other ways of supporting each other, and find appropriate twenty-first-century versions of them. And just as the COVID-19 pandemic is the latest iteration of the periodic plagues that have occurred throughout history, so it can spur a new era for care. The phrase 'mutual-aid' used to be relegated to political theory texts and activist circles, but during the height of coronavirus, it became part of the everyday lexicon of our frightening new world. Tens of thousands of mutual-aid groups sprang up, including the one in my mum's neighbourhood. There were so many that in both the UK and the USA, new umbrella organisations were established to support, resource and enable these groups. Media as diverse as the *New York Times* and *Pivot*, the magazine of the Chartered Professional Accountants of Canada, ran articles about the phenomenon. It was suddenly not only *possible* to get someone to drop groceries to my mother's door, but *acceptable* too. 'In my area in London, we have had so many [mutual-aid groups] that we've spun off down to street level,' one Londoner told journalist Rebecca Solnit for the *Guardian*. 'Our two-street collective has done shopping, picked up medicines, created an Easter-egg-in-the-window hunt for kids – all to help one another.' Another explained: 'Hackney in London has all the usual stuff, like grocery-buying and support, plus people are sourcing donated phones for people in hospital, laptops for kids who need them to access home learning, and cars for healthcare staff redeployed to the makeshift COVID-19 hospital.'[14]

In relation to her own work – and the same is true for mutual-aid networks, too – Cottam describes a 'model of abundance'. Unlike existing services, which are stretched and weakened by more people using them, these models grow stronger as more people become involved, because there are more hands on deck, more time available, more ideas, more bonds, more money. 'This is the most powerful inversion of all,' she explains in her book. 'If the critical resource is relationships, then the more people taking part, the stronger the service. Open the floodgates, bring everybody in: the more, the merrier.'

Many of the COVID-19 mutual-aid societies provide perfect examples of a new (or remembered) way of meeting our needs. Because they're rooted in equality and cooperation, they don't divide members into independent or dependent, able or disabled. Instead, they recognise our essential condition as Nussbaum's 'both capable and needy'. They're another way of nurturing 'generalised reciprocity', a concept we encountered in Chapter 4, which occurs when we give without an immediate expectation of receiving something in return. In that chapter, it was applied to families that went beyond bio-legal conventions. Here, we can see it stretched and broadened, turning from something sited in kinship relations to an atmospheric property, all around us, shaping our lives. There are so many ways in which this would help us with our care crisis – but also just with our lives in general.

First, it prevents the government from being our sole source of support. When it's the only place from which we can seek help, we're highly vulnerable to political changes. Scottish politician Jamie Stone recounted the following incident in a speech in parliament. He was holding a constituency clinic – a kind of open meeting in which constituents can bring their problems to their political representative – when a man in his early sixties came to see him. The man was living on a very low pension while caring for his mother, who was bedridden and incontinent. He was determined, he told Stone, not to put his mother into a home, because she'd looked after him all his life, so now it was his turn to do the same for her. The man began to cry in front of Stone as he explained what had provoked his visit: his mother had been given an allowance of four adult diapers each day, but this had suddenly been reduced to three. 'I'm not in my first youth,' the man said, as he broke down in front of the politician. 'I'm not as young as I was. It's the bed linen. It's nighties. I can't cope with this. I can't cope. I'm desperate.'[15]

This poor man was at the whim of whoever had reduced his allowance, and of his representative, who in this case – thankfully – was compassionate and resolved to sort it out for him. It's a story that shows the risks of being reliant on people over whom you have no real power. It's also a very practical example of why mutual-aid models matter. I know all about adult incontinence diapers. I know that when someone dies, leaving almost two dozen unused ones behind, you can't return them. There are rules against them being sent to someone else who needs them, even though they're individually wrapped and sealed, and so are perfectly safe. An economy of abundance would have ways to change this – to see me at my mum's, her bed horribly empty, crowded by supplies that wouldn't be needed anymore, and turn that man's hardship and my helplessness into mutual support.

And we wouldn't have to navigate the maddening bureaucracies that come with government care provision. Any caregiver will tell you that an enormous amount of time and energy is expended on this, which would be better spent on either self-care or care of their loved one. 'We have to apply for services,' Line explains to me from her native Norway. 'If we didn't do that, nothing would happen . . . And we always say, you have to have a first [class] degree [from] law school to fill all the forms and the application. And it's a fight with the system to get the right amount of help for your child . . . Those who shout the loudest, they get the best.'

Josie, all the way on the south-west coast of England, has similar thoughts. She thinks the government needs to offer people much more support, but that caregivers 'shouldn't have to go looking for it, because they're so drained and so tired from what they do every day'. Although Josie is speaking about government-provided services, a well-established local mutual-aid network could fulfil at least some of the role she describes. Circle's staff purposefully reached out to the people in its vicinity, explaining the project to them and enabling their involvement, but always directed and steered by its members. The members have the power; the paid staff are there to serve their self-government. Mutual-aid networks during COVID-19 put flyers through neighbourhood doors, set up websites and social media groups for local people, and created dedicated phone lines. It's all possible, though as we'll see in Chapter 8, it needs governments to behave differently in terms of money, power and regulations before it can be achieved.

Perhaps most crucially of all, these sorts of localised, self-governed networks can respond more quickly when an urgent care need occurs. Almost every caregiver I spoke with worried about what would happen if they themselves were sick or had an accident. Most were getting by with shockingly little practical help from people in their local area or family. Some caregivers create emergency plans in case they're suddenly incapacitated. Katy tried to make one, which required her to name two people who could replace her if need be. 'I've got some really good neighbours that'll help if he [her husband Mark] falls over and I need someone to help me get him up. A neighbour cuts my lawn for me, which is so nice. She doesn't even need to be asked . . . So I've got a small support network – I could walk up and down my road and knock on doors to ask for help with things if I have to. So that's reassuring, but it's not formalised at all,' she told me. She felt strange asking people to obligate themselves in the way the emergency plan required. In a society with a stronger concept of mutual-aid, where localised networks were the norm and everyone had experienced stepping in to help others and being helped themselves, this might be different. The realisation that she couldn't think of who to write down on her emergency plan was 'eye-opening', Katy says. 'You need networks of people you can rely on to do this bit or that bit, but I couldn't think of two people who would be available or able to do everything. Probably, it would have to be ten people who all did a tiny little bit of the whole.' Mutual-aid networks, Circle and OWCH are all ways of providing this capacity – and there are many more.

A plague of commitments

There's a deep and painful irony to observe here. We valorise individualist freedom as if it's strong, but it's incredibly frail. When our time of ease has passed, our once-lauded freedom flips swiftly into abject vulnerability. We are alone and needy, without sufficient support. Clearly, we must live consciously interdependent lives if we want to live well. But there's a risk to this. If we live embedded in a web of relations, we may become nothing but a servant to other people's needs. As we saw in Chapter 2, women especially risk being defined solely by their caring relationships. Our lives might become 'a plague of commitments',[16] our ability to make our own choices time-limited until chance makes a loved one sick or injured. A billiard ball maybe hard and alone, but at least it determines its own shape and trajectory.

It may feel compelling to run away from these truths. It may seem appropriate to condemn this relegation of human potential to the repetitive drudgery of caregiving, as Beauvoir might see it. But don't. Because the inescapable truth is this: human life *is* a plague of commitments. At some times, those commitments are greater, and at others lesser. Some people manage to dodge them, always at the expense of others. And plague is an apt word for what's happening in the world right now, because caregiving is so hard, so life-destroying, and, like being plagued by something, it causes continual trouble and distress. In recognising our fundamental unfreedom, we don't condone the hardship of care. Instead, it's a call to action, to organise ourselves, our communities and our political arenas in ways that alchemise those commitments from crushing plague to supportive web.

We began this chapter by understanding that we are not free. The human condition is bound by love and obligation. Our world is what academic Maria Puig de la Bellacasa describes as 'a thick mesh of relational obligation'.[17] Solving the care crisis is not, at its root, about shifting money or inspecting the quality of care homes, though both those aspects matter too. It's a question of dethroning the falsehood of the free individual and replacing it with a conception of the self that's embedded in relationships, whose autonomy is predicated on their support. We cannot expect to live a life entirely in pursuit of our own projects, but instead one that better resembles a duet between those ambitions and the requirements of love. This isn't just a political issue. It is painfully, cavernously personal. My mum's life – her death, too – would have been remarkably improved by living in a world that included local, self-governed and loving networks of support in it. So would my life. I want that different future for you.

CHAPTER 7

On Work:
Breadwinners or Caregivers

'Why should I let the toad work
Squat on my life?'
– Philip Larkin[1]

From the outside, my life looked like it was going well in summer 2019. A year before, I'd got a job with a not-for-profit I really respected. Most of my roles until then had been in rundown offices – one even had a rodent infestation – but this was situated in a beautiful modern building with huge windows and lots of plants. To top it off, I'd just signed the contract for my first book, putting me firmly on the path to realising my lifelong dream of being an author. And most importantly of all, my mum was in remission from cancer. At last, the years of chemotherapy and bad prognoses might be behind us. I chatted with colleagues as we started our day, clearing emails and preparing for meetings. My phone rang. I knew before I looked at the screen whose name would be there. It was my mum's, and although it was only Wednesday, it was the second time that week she'd called me urgently while I was at work, the fifth time in a fortnight. I stepped into the corridor, steadied myself, and clicked 'answer'. She made the scared sound I'd come to expect.

That phase of being her caregiver ought to have been straightforward. There were no more ravaging treatments or weekly blood tests. Finally, after a donor stem-cell transplant and even more chemo, the lymphoma had been beaten into submission. She was, apparently, 'better'. When I told people that she was in remission, there were sighs of relief on my behalf, sometimes hugs. The battle was over – we could lay down our weapons, allow our bruised hearts to venture out from behind the protective walls we'd built around them. Except that this 'better' looked suspiciously like sickness. The transplant had caused 'graft versus host disease', in which the donated cells attack the host body. Multiple types of chemo had also wrecked her body. Movies about people 'beating' cancer tend to omit the devastation of chronic symptoms and conditions caused by contemporary medical interventions, and I can see why: instead of remission being our triumphant denouement, we remained stuck in the suffocating repetition of fevers, vomiting spates, incontinence and potentially fatal infections. Several of those infections had already led to hospitalisation, even though for a healthy person they'd have been barely a sniffle.

My sister had her second child that summer, so she was largely unavailable. Sadly, my mother's older brother had died of brain cancer at the start of the year. Her two remaining siblings seemed to be understandably keen on her remission affording a pause in the list of family tragedies. I was trying to live at my own place again, but it wasn't working very well. I'd given up leaving the house without spare underwear, a clean top and my toothbrush in my work bag, because I couldn't predict where I'd be each night. Would it be at my house, where I lived with housemates and tried to pretend my life looked like any other thirty-something's? Or at my mum's, my feet propped on the side of her bed, watching her lie there listlessly, checking her temperature every half an hour and trying to convince her she'd feel better soon? Or in a chair covered with squeaky blue plastic, hospital smells pricking my nose, reaching out a tired hand to mute the drip machines that seemed to beep constantly? I had no idea from one day to the next in which evening scene I'd find myself. All I knew was that my life was no longer my own. I coped with the chaos by smoking cigarettes. I'd smoke one, then feel better for a few minutes before the sensation of freefalling caught up with me again. Then I'd count down until I could smoke the next one, my hand clasping it like a rope above an abyss. If this had been the first time I was living in a state of emergency, I might have cruised through it, steely and stoic. But her sickness had gone on too long; my steel and stoicism were all burned up and broken. I cried as I shoved my stuff into my bag yet again and left the office, telling my colleagues I'd be back online from my mum's as soon as possible, and would catch up then.

An hour later, I was at her house, climbing the stairs to find her in her bed, lying in miserable silence. 'I thought you'd never come,' she said querulously, even though she knew the length of my journey from work to her house. But I didn't need to point that out. This had happened enough times now for me to know what she really meant: she was afraid and lonely. I did what I did every time: checked her temperature, dispensed paracetamol, applied a cool, damp flannel to her forehead, coaxed her to drink more water, held her hand. Most times, her symptoms were just a passing and enigmatic fever, combined with a mental state of dejection and loneliness, despite her refusal to live with anyone else formally. The physical symptoms usually passed once she'd been persuaded to take pills and drink fluids. But, every so often, the fever would keep creeping up, and we'd end up back in hospital. There was no way of predicting which outcome it would be, so I had no way of organising my life. And every time one of these urgent calls happened, once she was calmer at home or we were ensconced in a hospital room, I'd open my laptop to try to catch up on work, feeling half guilty not to be giving her my full attention, and half guilty to be working in such a state of distraction.

Much has been written about the guilt of the working parent, especially the working mother. I understand the importance of highlighting working mothers' experiences and providing appropriate support, not least because I was brought up by a working mother who felt social opprobrium about her choice to prioritise her career. But the total absence of caregivers from this conversation about work and responsibilities in the home is immensely frustrating when you're in the latter category. It adds to your sinking loneliness, to be so thoroughly unnoticed by society. And yet, a lot of our experiences are the same as parents – exhaustion, needing to work part-time, lower earnings, aching guilt at not being everywhere at once, etc. – so it would surely be better for everyone if the conversation about care and work was widened to encompass *all* who provide care. This is especially true given that eldercare will be the new childcare, as the trends explored in Chapter 1 demonstrate. In fact, many people will be caring for sick older adults longer than they cared for their offspring. Already today, in the USA, over a sixth of working people are also caregivers for elderly or disabled family members,[2] and more than half of them are working full-time. I was one of 3.7 million working caregivers in England and Wales.[3] Despite this prevalence, very little attention is given to the difficulties of juggling work with the kind of care I'm talking about.

The failure to recognise that many workers are also caregivers manifests in high absence rates as people take unplanned time off to provide this hidden form of care. The toll of trying to do everything without sufficient support harms their health, further increasing rates of absence. I was ill more times than I can count because there was never enough opportunity for me to rest and truly get well; I was always either needed at home or catching up on work. Like many, I reduced my working days, first to four, then to three, but it wasn't enough. I was trying to squeeze too much work into too little time, while my body and mind buckled under the strain of my circumstances. And remember, care is erratic and unpredictable. The sickness of your loved one doesn't care whether today is a 'work day' or a 'day off' earmarked for care. This is where the bodily reality of care rears its head again. Kids get sick temporarily and have accidents, but on the whole, they can be bundled up each morning and shipped off to school for a predictable number of hours – once they're a certain age, anyway. The implicit assumption of that predictability was evident during 2020 and 2021, when schools shut entirely or operated erratic hours because of COVID-19. Parents were, understandably, shocked, overwhelmed, exhausted and unable to work. While I don't take the energy required to look after children (and home school them, too) lightly at all, it strikes me that this sudden extreme situation is, in reality, very similar to normal life for caregivers, regardless of pandemics.

Care isn't an occasional interruption of an otherwise relatively steady pattern of life. For many types of long-term illness, it's the inverse – interruption is the constant. It's almost impossible to plan or predict what will happen from one day to the next. This is partly because of the erratic nature of lots of sicknesses and impairments, and also because if your loved one is having medical treatment, you have no control over when appointments are scheduled. There will be a short-notice appointment for bloods to be taken on a Monday, chemo on the Thursday, a consultant appointment the following Wednesday, a sudden scan required that Friday, and so on. For parents, the odds are that interruption isn't the norm, much as parenting is chaotic, because most days they'll be able to drop their child at nursery or school (notwithstanding extortionate fees at pre-school ages in many countries). Their child will be cared for during a set number of hours, several days a week. That expected predictability is why the pandemic and its school closures were such a shock – parents were accustomed to a regular routine which meant other people were looking after their children while they worked. But even outside pandemic times, this isn't what happens for caregivers because, conventionally and ethically, we must consider the autonomy of the adults for whom we care more than we might do with children. This means that mostly, we don't get to send our sick loved ones to external centres to be cared for, not unless that's what they expressly want. It would also likely be unsafe for many conditions. Neither parenting nor caregiving are easy – the point isn't to create a competition of which is harder, but rather to note their distinctness so that we can choose appropriate solutions.

One day in summer 2020, I was working in my mum's kitchen while she lay in bed upstairs, as she was almost always doing by then. I looked out of the window and saw that the sun was out, the sky a bright, clear blue. It was the first glorious weather in a fortnight. For all I knew, it would be the last sunny day she'd be well enough for me to take her out in her wheelchair. There was a café near her house that I'd been hoping to push her along to. We could sit outside and have tea, maybe even a slice of cake. I could watch her enjoy something for once. I knew then I had to resign, and quickly. I couldn't spend any more hours looking at my emails when I should be tending to her. My experience – the exhausting attempt to juggle work and care, the guilt of feeling you're letting down both sides, the reduction in hours and related loss of pay, the tears, the tension headaches, the depleted immune system and the eventual resignation – are stereotypical for the caregiver. I regret not quitting sooner.

My mum loved flowers, and she had a few pots of red geraniums on her bedroom balcony. She'd asked me to water them one afternoon. I forgot, until I was about to leave for work the next day and was too exhausted to do it. By the time she died, a handful of weeks after I'd resigned from my job, the flowers were shrivelled, darkened, their stalks drooping reproachfully over the sides of the tubs. I still think about those geraniums. That she had to look at them like that in her dying days, because I'd been too tired from work to water them. Months later, I was vacuuming her bedroom, the furniture gone, her things gone too, only dust tracing the outlines of where they'd been. Her house had been sold – not *her* house, then, *a* house. And in the corner, greyed with dust, a dead curling geranium petal.

Losing our sense of self

If we'd encountered Line and Katy twenty years ago, we'd have met two women in their thirties, enjoying their chosen profession of teaching. Today, they're in their fifties, and one remains a teacher while the other has had, she tells me, no choice but to create a different identity.

It's evident from the way Line's expression broadens and clears as she describes her work that she gets a great deal of satisfaction from teaching. She's also found that her home life as a caregiver for Tarjei, who's aphasic, has benefits for her profession: 'I have a good connection with my pupils. I can read them. I can see when they're not happy, and if they're sad, and when they need me to stop in the hallway and just [say], "Come on, let's talk. What's the problem?" I've learned how to read people . . . it's really satisfying.' She still plays concerts and goes on tour sometimes, too. Line has been able to keep working throughout Tarjei's life because of the services available from her municipality, as well as some help from Tarjei's sisters and, currently, an employer who's accommodating. Tarjei goes to a free day care centre while Line and her husband are at work, and has two types of respite care each month, one for a week, and one for five days, which can be spread throughout the month as suits their schedules. When he's away, Line's either touring or sleeping. She also has thirty-five days of paid sick leave each year – ten more than is standard for other Norwegians because she has a disabled child – in addition to paid holiday. Even so, she tells me she's 'constantly tired', because caring for Tarjei has been 'like having really small children for twenty-two years . . . he didn't sleep until he was fifteen. I was up ten times at night and then getting up in the morning and going to work.' Earlier in Tarjei's life, this extreme situation meant she had to take long periods of sick leave, of a month or two at a time. Under Norwegian law, her job was kept for her to return when she was strong enough.

In contrast to Line, Katy is no longer a teacher. She went part-time around fifteen years ago, when she was helping her mum to care for her terminally ill father. Then Mark, her husband, was diagnosed with motor neurone disease, and she had to leave her job entirely. Her situation differs to Line's in many ways, not least that caring for a spouse is different to caring for a child. Mark is Katy's equal, so understandably, the idea of sending him somewhere each day, as a parent might a child, feels ill-fitting. When I ask her what would help, she tells me: 'My husband would have to be accepting of someone else coming into the house . . . he wouldn't be accepting of it at the moment. I've got to be led by him. I can't inflict this on him.'

For Katy, her understandable wish to respect Mark's preferences and the erratic nature of his disease makes a standard working life impossible. 'There'd be times when he'd have a choking fit or a fall at work, and I'd have to then get him,' Katy explains, when I ask why she left her job. 'It took away a level of added worry to leave work, because at least I didn't have to worry about my job as well. Maybe there are other jobs I could have done if I had a really understanding boss and colleagues.'

Katy has channelled her industrious nature into creating a new campaign for the rights of caregivers. It is, in her own words, a new identity she's built, having had no choice but to leave her previous self behind.

Our work isn't our sole source of identity. Indeed, for billions of people, work is nothing more than daily toil to survive. But for the lucky in our global economy, work is a site of purpose, a place where we pursue self-expression and feel like small parts of a greater whole. At work, if we're fortunate, we forge relationships, explore our capabilities, and tap into our creativity. We can be known as an adult in our own right, rather than solely as the family role we play, and we can be respected for skills and knowledge beyond the domestic. We also care about work because of our cultural morality. Being unemployed is judged as equal to being lazy or idle, immoral and unacceptable. Care theorist Professor Joan Tronto has written that the 'work ethic' is treated as a public good, and that the cultural assumption is that the responsible, morally upstanding person meets their needs through work. It's the underlying premise of arguments against welfare and denigrations of those on the dole. 'This image of what constitutes responsible human action misses entirely the [caregiving] that is necessary to keep human society functioning,' she writes.[4] In this world, where responsible human action is supposed to mean going to work each day, and where care is omitted, overlooked and made invisible, the inability to work because of care can crush people's self-esteem. While there are interesting arguments being made about how we can undo this moralistic notion of toil, for now it remains the case that many caregivers want to work, and that our failure to enable that is deeply harmful.

It's obvious caregivers feel this way because many keep working even when they're utterly exhausted from their dual responsibilities, and even when they are in economic circumstances where they could work less or stop entirely. We've already met Line, who's doing just that, and Safa's mum is another good example. Safa is the eldest of four children, all of whom go to different schools, so they have to be dropped off at different locations each day. Her father owns a restaurant and works 'pretty much six days a week', so her mum is left doing almost everything at home, except for the bits of caring Safa does instead. Despite this enormous load and generally being 'very stressed', her mum still works part-time as a teaching assistant because she enjoys it. Safa thinks if her sister needed less support, her mum would like to work more. The organisation Working Families surveyed parents of disabled children, and found that ninety per cent of those who weren't currently in paid work wanted to be.[5] Feminist economist Nancy Folbre uses the term 'care penalty' to capture the economic disadvantages caused by having caring responsibilities. It's commonly used to refer to the loss in income, in pension savings and other benefits, which we've already explored. But it's a loss that goes much deeper than money alone, important as that is. We need to think of this penalty as reaching into every part of a working caregiver's life, into their very sense of self.

The work world forgets that we're humans as well as labourers. Consequently, care is often treated as a sector in which some people work, and others don't. You're a hairdresser? You don't do care; you do hair. You're a lawyer? Care's not relevant for you. And so on. Recall Dr Allard's interviewees in Chapter 5, who were interrogated by employers about why they needed to provide care and have time off their jobs to do so. When we think of care as something done by paid care workers as part of a discrete economic sector, it's easy to forget that it's a practice of life, or, to use that term from Chapter 2, a 'species activity'. Yes, it is some people's job, but, unlike hairdressing or law, it's also everyone's responsibility.

Ubasute or Uber?

Political theorist Professor Nancy Fraser has pointed out that within capitalism lies a deep contradiction. This economic system relies on activities that nurture and reproduce human life, while at the same time it chases after profit in such a way that destabilises those necessary activities.[6] Over time, she explains, this jeopardises the necessary social conditions of the capitalist economy, creating a crisis. If we take Fraser's explanation as a prognosis of what's to come regarding care, then she's right to predict danger. Skyrocketing care needs, too few people to provide that care and insufficient support for them will wreak havoc on our economies, not to mention our personal lives and wellbeing. We could solve this by no longer considering it morally necessary to care for the sick, elderly or impaired. In that scenario, we simply don't care anymore; people die when their usefulness to our economy is outstripped by their dependence. It would mean a revival of ancient customs, like *ubasute* in Japan. Literally translating as 'abandoning an old woman', infirm relatives were allegedly carried to a remote place, like a mountain, and left there to die.[7] The ancient people of the island Keos, in the Aegean Sea, are alleged to have required all people over the age of sixty to take their own lives in order to ensure there was enough food to go round for the younger people.[8] This scenario would require a complete cultural overhaul and, presumably, it's not the kind of world we want to inhabit.

More likely, this crisis tendency will be patched up with 'solutions' that do little to address the underlying causal tension of work versus care. In fact, these quick fixes are already here. When Harvard graduate Sheila Lirio Marcelo had her second son, her parents came to the US from the Philippines to support her and her husband. Then one day, her father had a heart attack while carrying his grandson up the stairs. 'In that moment,' she explained in a media interview, 'everything changed. I wasn't thirty yet, but I was sandwiched between caring for my children and an ailing parent.'[9] Her struggle to find paid care workers inspired her to create Care.com: essentially, Uber for care workers.

Her platform solves the 'problem' of care so that kin can go to work as usual, offloading it on to other women, all in the name of keeping the wheels of commerce turning. 'Without care, people can't work,' its website explains, and work is, apparently, the most important function of all. Care.com was one of the winners from the pandemic, as corporations sought to keep their employees at work despite the sudden care load on their shoulders. Amazon announced a new 'family care benefit through Care.com to 650,000 full- and part-time Amazon and Whole Foods Market employees in the U.S.'.[10] This follows Fraser's 'Universal Breadwinner' model, which we encountered in Chapter 2. In this approach, everyone is a breadwinner, and mechanisms like day care are put in place to keep workers at their desks and production lines, no matter what's happening at home. In practice, it looks like prioritising work and offloading care. But care can't truly be offloaded. We still need to participate in the care of our loved ones in all the ways described already – arranging, overseeing and vetting the care service, filling in the gaps and being able to cover urgent changes. Then, of course, there's the idea that we may *want* to be with sick loved ones.

Instead of quick fixes that focus more on what's good for business than what's good for humans, we've got to have a conversation about *the right to provide care ourselves*, at least some of the time, and making jobs fit for that reality. This third option doesn't involve reintroducing senicide or prioritising work over care. Rather, it means that *all* jobs need to be appropriate for caregivers because we're *all* going to be caring. Care shifts from being a *women's* problem to being a *human* problem, from being a *sector* to being a *species activity*. We've heard of the hunter-gatherer model of the pre-agricultural past, of the breadwinner-housewife ideal of industrialisation – today, we need to become *provider-caregivers*, humans who provide for their kin materially, probably by working, and also perform care.

The three changes we need

Time to work less

Our time is organised by work. We speak of having a 'lifetime', but arguably, 'worktime' would be more appropriate, given how we spend our lives. It is common to work five days per week, and that time is usually batched together in a clump with 'free time' on the weekend, when you're supposed to do everything else. I've always found this a strange way to organise our lives. I remember getting my first nine-to-five job and being completely bemused by how I was meant to do all the other bits of life – the admin, the dentist appointments and so on – when the surgeries and offices I needed were mostly open when I was at work. It doesn't make sense! And it makes even less sense for the human of the future, the provider-caregiver. How can we change our apportionment of time to meet the needs of that future homo sapiens?

Iceland has part of the answer. Between 2015 and 2019, Reykjavík City Council and the national government tested shorter working weeks with no loss in pay.[11] More than 2,500 workers at a range of workplaces, including schools, hospitals and offices, took part. Researchers described the experiments as an 'overwhelming success' – productivity remained the same or improved, while workers reported feeling less stressed, found their health had improved, and said they had more time to spend with families and for domestic tasks. In 2022, trials of four-day weeks were taking place in the UK, USA, Spain, Canada, Australia, New Zealand and more.[12] Although it feels like something as natural as trees and water, the conventional five-day week hasn't actually been convention for very long. Nineteenth- and early-twentieth-century campaigning by organised labourers, and the impact of the Great Depression, are what got us here. In fact, the USA only officially adopted a five-day system in 1932.[13] Change was possible then, and it is now. Today, activists, academics and business people are reviving the call for a shorter working week on the grounds that it could reduce carbon footprints, improve mental and physical wellbeing, create more good jobs and give us more time for leisure. And, crucially, it would mean more time available for care, enabling the provider-caregiver of the future to thrive. There is, then, a compelling array of reasons why a shorter working week should be introduced. Part of its genius is that it would be the standard model of working time. Today, many women already work shorter weeks because of caring responsibilities, but this has entrenched gender inequality rather than moving us towards an equal provider-caregiver approach. Women who work part-time are judged negatively – they're seen as taking the 'mommy track' as Nancy Fraser called it, and as not being sufficiently committed or ambitious. Without changing *all* jobs to require fewer hours, we end up with stigma and gender injustice.

This seemed common sense when I first learned about the

shorter working week campaigns, but then I discovered the proof of it: two cases from Scandinavia show us precisely why it's important we change all jobs, rather than just relying on women choosing to work fewer hours and taking the subsequent hit in pay. The first case takes us back to 1970s Sweden. While ABBA were ushering in a new dawn of pop, the women's movement was campaigning for a reduction in the working day from eight hours to six. Instead of meeting this demand, the government introduced a measure that allowed parents of young children to reduce their work days to six hours, losing the pay from the removed hours while standard work days remained eight hours long. Mothers tended to be the workers who took the former option, with fathers more likely to work full-time.[14] Because it was applied asymmetrically, the policy failed at achieving gender equality.

At the same time, a little to the west, academics were setting up an experiment in Norway that would take decades to publish its results. The Work-Sharing Couples Project was led by sociologist Erik Grønseth of the University of Oslo, who was a long-standing critic of male-breadwinner family arrangements. Sixteen couples were selected, all with children below school age. Rather than following the male-breadwinner model, these young families attempted to share both working and caring roles, becoming provider-caregivers. Decades later, researchers followed up with the sons of those families, seeking to compare the generations and see whether the gender-neutral approach to activities had stuck. It hadn't. The sons' families lived in 'neo-traditional' arrangements: 'Both partners had paid work, and both were involved in the care of their children, but the men worked slightly more and their wives slightly less, and there was a corresponding gender division of household work.'[15] Without making changes to working hours mandatory and universal, we can't create the conditions necessary for the provider-caregiver to become the norm.

Despite the hope that a shorter working week is on the horizon thanks to successful trials and tireless campaigning, there's one glaring problem. Many arguments made in favour of a shorter working week focus on there being no loss in productivity or profit. But if winning shorter working weeks for everyone is contingent on keeping productivity and profits at the same level as before, we'll create a two-tiered work world in which 'knowledge workers' are more likely to get shorter hours and manual workers still toil for longer. This merely amends the same narrative that brought us to the brink of a care catastrophe in the first place: work trumps care, productivity trumps humanity. To be available to all, not just the middle classes, the provider-caregiver model requires work and care to stand as equals, and for that equality to be enshrined in law. This, in turn, necessitates deep changes to the very way we think.

Consider statistics on work and caregiving. A Gallup-Healthways poll reported that because seventeen per cent of US full-time workers also act as caregivers, there are 126 million 'missed workdays each year'.[16] How many 'caredays' are missed because caregivers are also acting as full-time workers? We don't even have the word 'careday' in our vocabulary. Likewise, a MetLife study reports that: 'The cost of informal caregiving in terms of lost productivity to U.S. businesses is $17.1 to $33 billion annually.'[17] What are the costs of caregivers being unable to perform the tasks their loved ones need? This isn't a fluffy question. Research shows that the more stressed the caregiver, the worse the health outcomes for the care recipient, and, as we saw in Chapter 1, caregivers themselves are storing up all manner of physical, financial and social problems when they're having to burn the candle at both ends.

The short-story version of a working life

'I felt like, for the first time in my life, it was someone putting words to my experience and making it important as a political issue, not something that you have to deal with on your own,' Dr Camille Allard explains when I ask her why she's chosen care as her academic focus. She goes on:

> When I was a young teenager, I was ill for quite a long time and, at that time, we were living in the countryside, so the nearest hospital was fifty kilometres away. So my mum had to drive me every time. When I was really bad, I needed help for everything. I couldn't be left on my own. So that really had an impact on my mum; she couldn't work . . . And then when I started recovering, my mum had to start caring for my grandmother, who got breast cancer. So you see, I could really see that my mum was always caring for someone.

Like many women who've decided to study aspects of care, and like me writing this book, Dr Allard was drawn to the topic because she could see it shaping her life and the lives of the women around her. In Dr Allard's case, her focus on working caregivers is highlighting the plight of billions who go over-looked around the world.

To raise new humans and to care for those who need sup-port after infancy, we need to take leaves of absence from our jobs over the course of our lives. This is a familiar idea when it comes to parenting but, given the trends outlined in Chapter 1, our attention needs to turn to the kind of pattern appropriate for an ageing, chronically unwell population. Our expectations of our working lives must change. Rather than the ideal of continuous presence, we need to normalise repeated absences of varying lengths as people deal with emergencies, illnesses and the increased needs of loved ones. This would stop caregivers feeling, like I did, that they're trapped in an endless merry-go-round of guilt, always letting down work or home, unable to be everything for everybody. Instead of our work lives being like continuous narratives, they can become a series of short stories, punctuated by care. Employers must expect to have job applicants who've taken career breaks, instead of balking at empty years on a CV. Intelligent employers will realise those years aren't empty at all, but are filled with lessons and skills, like those learned by Line, who is now far better attuned to her pupils because of caring for Tarjei.

And for shorter breaks within the same job, we need legal rights to paid leave if we're going to get to the provider-caregiver ideal. According to Dr Allard, there are four criteria necessary for an ideal care-leave policy. First, we need to be paid when we take time off to care. When caregiver leave does exist today, is often unpaid, or so poorly paid as to be unfeasible for most workers. Second, there needs to be flexibility in how and when that leave is taken – you need to be able to take two hours, or a week, or a few days, etc. This responds to the unpredictability of caregiving already discussed. Third, Dr Allard says we need to be asking employees what they want, because different types of work will need different provisions. Dr Allard is of French origin. In France, trade unions remain strong. She views collective agreements, negotiated by workplace unions, as the best way to determine the specifics of each employer's care-leave policy. And fourth, job protection is vital, meaning workers can take care leave and come back to the same job, at the same status and the same pay, without being penalised. Many countries already have this in place for maternity leave.

Leave for family care has been big news in the USA in recent years, helped into the headlines by the Biden presidency and the COVID-19 pandemic. The Family Medical Leave (FML) Act of 1993 has provided leave allowances for the past three decades. In theory, it means a US worker can get twelve weeks of unpaid leave per year to provide care. In practice, it's a very restricted right. FML applies only to employees who have worked for their employer for at least twelve months; have worked for at least 1,250 hours in that time; and who work at a physical work location where at least fifty employees work within seventy-five miles of that location.[18] Try saying that five times fast. As if that wasn't enough restriction, only private-sector employers with fifty or more employees across all their locations are covered, though public agencies are covered regardless of their size. The US Department of Labor has analysed how FML is working and who tends to use it. In its 2020 review, they found that forty-one per cent of private-sector employees weren't at worksites large enough to be eligible.[19] Even if you do meet the eligibility factors, FML is only applicable for an immediate family member, defined as a parent, spouse or child – an idea of the 'family' that is outdated, as we saw in Chapter 4. And because FML is unpaid, lower-wage workers are less likely to take it.

Thankfully, some states have created laws with better provisions. In California, a paid leave programme introduced in 2004 has been celebrated, not least because it's reduced nursing home usage, 'likely because the policy gave workers sufficient flexibility to provide informal care to family members on the side'.[20] In New York, the recent Paid Family Leave Benefits Law allows employed New Yorkers to take up to ten weeks of paid leave annually in order to care for an elderly relative with a serious illness, which is defined to include a disability resulting from natural ageing. Wisely, the state allows people to take this however suits them, so they can take it all at once, in large chunks, or spread it out across the year, for example reducing their working days by one day per week.[21] President Biden's Build Back Better plan has sought to follow the lead of these states at a federal level by introducing paid caregiver leave nationwide.[22] Pay would replace earnings on a sliding scale, with lower-paid workers receiving a greater percentage of their income than higher earners. Introducing paid leave for caregivers undoes the paradox at the heart of our current caring models: today, we can be paid to look after someone else's kin, but not our own.

The UK fares no better – and, arguably, much worse – than the USA when it comes to caregivers and leave rights. Employees have a right to 'dependant leave', but this is unpaid and, crucially, only for emergencies. It's not useable 'if you knew about the situation beforehand', for example to take a child to a hospital appointment that was made in advance.[23] Think about how absurd that is. How does knowing in advance about an appointment make taking leave to accompany your loved one any less necessary? How far in advance counts? At the time of writing, the current government has committed to introducing a right to caregiver leave of just five days a year – without pay. Several European countries are doing better, although flaws abound. In her native France, Dr Allard tells me that caregivers now have paid leave for up to three months a year. She points out that it remains flawed because the compensation is too low, but 'it's a good advancement'. In the Netherlands, workers can take short-term care leave of up to ten days a year for seventy per cent of their wage. However, long-term care leave is unpaid.[24] Other countries, including Belgium and Germany, have leave especially for people with a terminally ill loved one.[25]

The European Union has recently introduced a requirement for member states to have a minimum of five days of caregivers' leave a year, but it doesn't have to be paid.[26] This tells us what's minimally acceptable, but what's at the other end of the scale? Where is our legal right to what we actually need?

Perhaps it's slow to materialise because care itself is absent from our human rights. Consider this: the UN Universal Declaration of Human Rights states clearly that 'everyone has the right to work'. What about the right to care for our loved ones? At best, we could argue that Article 16(3) of the Declaration covers this. It says: 'The family is the natural and fundamental group unit of society and is entitled to protection by society and the State.'

But this is far less effective than a simple statement that we each have *the right to provide care.* In 1948, when the Declaration was passed, this would have seemed an unnecessary provision. After all, women were supposed to be at home, providing that care for free. Why would the right to care need to exist? Today, without that right in place, a cascade of other omissions and constraints exist that make it almost impossible to become the provider-caregivers we need to be.

Earlier, in the examples of the Swedish six-hour day and the Norwegian Work-Sharing Couples Project, we saw that we must make changes mandatory and universal if our working patterns are to change and stay changed. The same principle applies to caregivers' leave. In the UK, shared parental leave was introduced in 2015. It allows two parents of a new child to share the leave they take for those early months between them. Specifically, they have fifty weeks to share. It was hailed as a step forward for gender equality, because men could now take more time for parenting – but that's not what's happened. Six years later, the government estimates only two to eight per cent of men eligible to take shared parental leave do so. In other words, women are still taking the most time off.[27] There is a solution, and one which has been proven to work. This is to make leave non-transferable – that is, you 'use it or lose it'. Sweden has already done the work for us. In 1974, it led the world by replacing gender-specific maternity leave with gender-neutral parental leave. Couples could take six months off work per child, with each parent entitled to half the days. A father could, however, sign over his share to the mother. By 1994, the failure of the policy was evident: ninety per cent of the leave that men could have taken was instead being signed over to the mothers. The following year, Sweden introduced the *pappamånad*, or 'daddy month'. Thirty days of the leave allowance was only allowed to be taken by fathers – they couldn't sign those days over to the mother. It was use it or lose it. Since then, leave allowances have increased so fathers now have ninety non-transferable days. By 2020, fathers were taking thirty per cent of the total number of days available to the couple, rather than the ten per cent they were taking prior to the change.[28] It's not good enough, but it's better.

Those findings pertain to parenting, so what does the equivalent look like for caregivers? Well, for parents caring for a disabled child, regardless of the child's age, a similar mechanism could be in place that apportions a certain amount of paid leave to each parent. For those who, like me, were caring for other relatives, there could be a paid 'use it or lose it' quota available for designated family members. So, for example, a brother, husband or close friend. Consider Karen's situation. She does the daily care for both her parents, despite the fractious relationship she has with her father, and while forgoing shifts at work. Her brother, meanwhile, does financial management for them, which fits in around his schedule and doesn't involve the emotional and physical toil of hands-on care. If there was an option to be paid to care for their parents, and both Karen and her brother had an allotted number of days to which they were legally entitled but could not transfer to anyone else, Karen would have a much stronger argument to call on her brother to play his part. They might both be provider-caregivers, instead of so much being on Karen's tired shoulders.

In an ideal world, we wouldn't need these kinds of mandatory measures. Gender and profit wouldn't shape and dictate life paths, and we'd all be living as provider-caregivers. But we don't live in that world, and there are duties to be shared: duties about raising and caring for humans; duties about love.

Control in our hands

Recall my situation in 2019, when my mum called me to her house frequently during working hours, and I cried as I left my office. If I'd been working from home the whole time, I wouldn't have lost time travelling to my mum's each time she had an emergency, and I would probably have been able to intervene in some of those emergencies earlier, keeping her calmer and healthier overall. I wouldn't have been crying, either. Each morning is a game of roulette for many caregivers – will today be a day when your father with dementia can remember how to make eggs, or when he leaves the frying pan on the heat and causes a kitchen fire? Trying to predict this as your eyes open in the morning is both impossible and stressful. So, while shorter working weeks will free up more time for care, and rights to paid leave will enable us to take time off work without impoverishing ourselves or facing stigma, if we are to tackle the erratic and unpredictable nature of caregiving and the ways in which it interrupts work, we need to go further. 'Flexible working' means a change from the 'standard' arrangement of working five days a week between nine and five. It includes things like part-time work, term-time-only work, job sharing, compressed working hours and remote working.[29] During the COVID-19 pandemic, many people were allowed to work from home for the first time, opening the door to more flexibility, at least in terms of location. Working from home is very helpful for caregivers. Remote working would mean you're there for whatever the day might bring; you are both workforce and careforce. However, remote working is only applicable to certain types of jobs. You can't be a cleaner or a factory worker from a distance. To avoid further entrenching a labour market that works really well for the middle classes with knowledge-orientated jobs and appallingly for everyone else, we need solutions that work for *all* types of work, as far as possible.

When governments use the term 'flexible' about work, they often mean flexibility that suits businesses, not workers. Under the administration of George W. Bush, 'flextime' was used to describe a proposal that would have exempted businesses from paying overtime under some circumstances.[30] Likewise, in many European countries, talk of 'flexible labour markets' has come to mean the ways in which employers treat their workforce as disposable commodities, hiring and firing at will. For some workers, 'flexibility' poses problems for organising care responsibilities, because it's used to mean an employer sends out shift schedules with little advance notice. Flexible working, then, really lives up to its name; it's a term bent to the will of its user, and that's not what we need. Instead, the provider-caregiver needs *control*. We need to have a say over our working schedules.

Some workers already have this kind of control; the ones at the top. This would work fine if caregiving discriminated by job seniority and income, but it doesn't. If we accept the factual condition that we're humans and have caring responsibilities regardless of where circumstance has placed us, we see that all workers need access to schedule control. Across Europe, the majority of employees have some access to work-schedule flexibility, but this hides wildly varied proportions depending on the country in question, along with constraints on the nature of that flexibility, to whom it's applicable, and the need for willingness on the part of employers.[31] The UK and a growing number of US states have introduced a 'right to request' flexible working, but this doesn't guarantee that request will be granted. And that's if you summon the courage to ask in the first place. As American lawyer and political commentator Anne-Marie Slaughter has explained in her book, *Unfinished Business: Women, Men, Work and Family*: 'In a work culture in which commitment to your career is supposed to mean you never think about or do anything else, asking for flexibility to fit your work and your life together is tantamount to declaring that you do not care as much about your job as your co-workers do.' We're either too cowed by a culture that depreciates care to ask for what we need, or we're like Oliver Twist going to the workhouse master to ask for a second portion of gruel. We hold out our hands, asking for the time we need to care for our loved ones, and await their denial.

Empty hands without legal rights

Our hands will remain empty without legal rights and protections for caregivers. Eldercare is the new childcare because of its increasing volume, but it's also catching up in terms of litigation. In the USA, discrimination cases about family responsibilities have increased dramatically. Between 1996 and 2005, there were only 873 such cases, but between 2006 and 2015, there were 3,223. That's an increase of 269 per cent. The majority of these were parental cases, but eldercare cases are rising. According to the Center for WorkLife Law, 'eldercare is the new frontier'.[32] Currently, the laws on caregiver discrimination in the workplace are patchy and often rely on 'association' provisions, meaning that we're protected because we have a known association with someone with a disability. This is the case under the USA's Americans with Disabilities Act 1990 and the UK's Equality Act 2010. This tangential protection may have seemed sensible when caregiving was a less common part of the working person's life, but in the provider-caregiver model of the future, it looks shockingly outdated. Caregivers need to be protected in their own right. Without this, we're left relying on employers' goodwill. People also need to know that these rights exist. When I was caring for my mum, I had assumed I had no legal protections, because 'caregiver' isn't one of the nine officially protected characteristics under the UK's Equality Act 2010. I'm sure I'm not alone.

Some employers are already moving towards a more balanced model, albeit always with an emphasis on what's best for the bottom line. Facebook introduced up to six weeks of paid leave to care for seriously ill relatives, and three days to care for family members dealing with short-term illness.[33] Northwestern University in Illinois provides access to specialist advisors so that employees have 'comprehensive support for the complexities of adult care resources, from choosing assisted living facilities to understanding financing options'.[34] But these examples aren't good enough. Most people don't work in the few organisations going further than the law.

Moreover, today many people are not *employees* at all. Contemporary capitalism is doing away with this category, because it's more costly than alternatives like 'independent contractors', to whom labour laws, protections and benefits often don't apply. It's a perfect example of what Nancy Fraser explained: capitalism undermines the very conditions of its own possibility. In the UK, false self-employment is a common scourge in precarious, low-paid sectors. In the USA, even some doctors are 'independent contractors'. Allowing companies to choose voluntarily whether to provide what caregivers need, and limiting those provisions to an ever-dwindling number of 'employees', isn't going to work. Instead, we need governments to introduce rights and protections in the workplace for caregivers, regardless of their employment status. In the US, the call for nationwide rights is gaining steam. The Time's Up Foundation, which tackles gender-based discrimination at work, has called for all workers to have access to a baseline of federally funded family and medical leave. In 2015, a roster of big names in business, including from Etsy, Lyft and Harvard Business School, published a call for benefits to be both portable and universal so that people can take them between various work scenarios and have access to them regardless of their employment status.[35] This fits with the short-story version of the provider-caregiver's career, understanding that we'll need to move around, change jobs, and stop and start work during our lives.

Time for employers to wake up

Until we get the laws we need, there are some practical steps employers could take right now, and should take for *all workers that contribute to their profit*, not just those they directly employ. The first step is to wake up. A 2019 Harvard Business School report examining how employers can support caregivers found substantial ignorance on the part of businesses. While over eighty per cent of working caregivers thought caregiving affected their productivity, only twenty-four per cent of employers thought caregiving influenced performance.[36] The report recommends companies begin by conducting a regular care census to understand its workforce's caregiving responsibilities. It also recognises the need to move forward from archaic assumptions about career paths being uninterrupted. Once employers have the data and understand the needs of their workers, what next? They can introduce a 'caregiver passport'.[37] This documents the discussions and agreements regarding a worker's caregiving needs, and can provide access to specialist support or benefits. It can also be updated much more quickly than going through a formal process, which is key when considering how care responsibilities fluctuate. As a spokesperson from one of the few UK organisations with this scheme in place explained: 'An employee with caring responsibilities may say, "This is what I need for the next year"; but often it's "This is what I need right now," and then in two weeks' time it's this, and actually, in a month's time it's this . . . and so I review things regularly, using that, and just make changes when I need to. So, it's quite a live thing.'[38] Not only is this well attuned to the reality of care, it also sounds infinitely less exhausting than having to formally update a boss about an ever-changing and upsetting situation. Believe me, caregivers are tired enough as it is.

Dystopic alternatives

Being a working caregiver in the world today is exhausting, hard and lonely. There's no culture of discussing this kind of care at work. Parents have photos of their adorable offspring on their desks. They share that they're leaving early to do the school run or to go to their kid's concert. I value camaraderie at work, but wish it was expanded to caregivers too. For us, this invisible careforce of a different kind, there are no photos, and if we raise why we're exhausted, why we're leaving early or arriving late, we're met with the sideways smile, imbued with that specific mix of sympathy and discomfort known so well to those of us initiated into the darker side of care. The work world has been designed for a strange version of the human being, one who has no duties outside their office, who may care for other people, but not so much that he needs to be with them if injury or illness occur.

In her bestselling 2012 book, palliative care worker Bronnie Ware recounted the top five regrets that dying people had shared with her. The second of these was: 'I wish I hadn't worked so hard.'[39] In one future, where we fail to institute the provider-caregiver model or give everyone a right to provide care, we'll meet the demands of our ageing, sick population using outsourced care from the likes of Care.com. The middle classes will be working hard in their well-paid jobs, regretting the time not spent with dying loved ones, occasionally allowing their own old-age loneliness to cross their minds, and the working classes will be caring for the middle classes' loved ones, in turn unable to be with their own. Regret will be the water in which we swim.

Alternatively, in the provider-caregiver future, we'll be recognised as humans, our love and care will be of equal importance to ideas about productivity and profit creation, and that importance will be enshrined in law.

CHAPTER 8

On Government:
Commoning the Horizon

'If to change ourselves is to change our worlds, and the
relation is reciprocal, then the project of history making
is never a distant one but always right here, on the borders of our sensing, thinking, feeling, moving bodies.'
                                   – J.K. Gibson-Graham[1]

In Charlotte Perkins Gilman's 1915 novella *Herland*, three young
men make an expedition to a land rumoured to be populated
solely by women. Herland is 'too pretty to be true', brimming
with flowers and fruit-bearing trees, dotted by small fountains
amongst pristine roads and palaces. Accordingly, most sickness
has been overcome, and though old age still occurs, the older
women are confoundingly 'in the full bloom of rosy health,
erect, serene, standing sure-footed and light as any pugilist'.
The narrating character, Vandyck Jennings, is scandalised to
learn that children aren't cared for by their biological mothers:

'But a mother's love—' I ventured.

She studied my face, trying to work out a means of clear explanation.

'You told us about your dentists,' she said, at length, 'those quaintly specialised persons who spend their lives filling little holes in other persons' teeth – even in children's teeth sometimes.'

'Yes?' I said, not getting her drift.

'Does mother-love urge mothers – with you – to fill their own children's teeth? Or to wish to?'

'Why no – of course not,' I protested. 'But that is a highly specialised craft. Surely the care of babies is open to any woman – any mother!'

Childcare is not a private, personal responsibility in Herland, but a public one. Vandyck Jennings' encounter illustrates the idea that how we organise our communities is not 'natural' but chosen. Speculative fiction reminds us of this, bringing playful imagination to soften ways of being that have become sclerotic. When we consider caregiving for the sick, elderly and infirm through this imaginative lens, what do we discover? A similar tussle comes into view, decades old, between the private and public sectors, and which should rightly 'own' care. Calls by some members of the 1970s feminist movement (see Chapter 2) and their political descendants today require care to become a public concern in the same way as unemployment – both are construed as social risks affecting livelihoods and needing the support of public coffers and collective arrangement. More recently, caregiving has been recast as a public issue by its inclusion under the rubric of 'infrastructure', notably by US President Joe Biden.[2] This has riled those who consider the term to mean something physically solid. Dictionaries are lobbed from each side of the semantic battle, some circumscribing infrastructure as solely physical, others as the basic systems and services needed for a country to work effectively, whether or not one can touch them with one's hand. US Senator Kirsten Gillibrand tweeted:

> Paid leave is infrastructure.
> Child care is infrastructure.
> Caregiving is infrastructure.[3]

This tweet provoked a flurry of derisory – and quite funny – responses:

'Botox and plastic surgery are infrastructure.'[4]

'Taco Tuesday is infrastructure!'[5]

'Ranch dressing is infrastructure.'[6]

Much like Vandyck Jennings, these Twitter users were reacting to care being pulled over the public/private border. They need not have been quite so perturbed; closer examination of the care-as-infrastructure narrative shows that, while it could create more public support for caregiving, it's usually legitimised by suggesting it'll keep more people (namely women) in paid work.[7] In a way, then, making care a public issue is part of shoring up the private realm of the market, rather than reconceptualising it as a general human good.

Conversely, we can find multiple attempts that try to shift care in the opposite direction, from public provision back into the private sphere. In Chapter 1, we encountered 'deinstitution-alisation', in which care homes and asylums were shut down in preference of poorly funded and executed 'care in the commu-nity', which really meant in the private home. More recently, a subtler sibling of this process has taken place: austerity-driven cuts to public spending have reduced government services available in many countries, increasing the responsibility held by private individuals and the family. This process has been a hot political topic in the UK for my entire adult life (I was twenty-two when the 2008 global financial crisis happened), and the impact of the tension between public and private provision of care is evident in the lives of the other caregivers we've met in these pages, too. Consider Line versus Ayesha, the former in Norway caring for Tarjei, with reams of (imper-fect) public support, the latter in Kathmandu, with absolutely nothing from the government. Or Eric and Karen, both in the USA, and both providing care privately but in different ways. In Eric's case, his care was supplemented by paid professionals provided through Scott's health insurance. So, Scott received care from two private sources: his husband and a private com-pany. In Karen's case, the private family (namely, her) is doing the work, for now. For me and Katy in England, the failure to see care as a public issue means there is no legal right for us to take time off work for caring responsibilities, as we saw in the previous chapter. We both felt we had to leave our jobs, our private pain finding no space in the public world. It's a frustrating battle that appears to happen at a level far above the everyday lives of normal people, but in fact shapes many of the hardest and most intimate moments of our lives. It's also a false battle, because neither the public nor the private realms hold the solution to our looming caregiving crisis.

We've seen in previous chapters why the private spheres of the market and the family can't be relied upon. As a load-bearing wall, the family as it's currently constituted can't support the weight of care – this is already the case, and given projections on chronic disease and old age, will only become increasingly true. It's frightening to truly understand this and what it will mean for the lives of countless people in the future. Paid care can't sufficiently reinforce family care. First, care bought from the market isn't financially feasible for everyone. Second, commercially driven care necessarily treats it like a factory production line, to the detriment of both its workforce and its customers. Robots may be useful for some tasks but, as we saw in Chapter 3, they're not a sufficient solution in themselves, and may well create more work for caregivers, not less, just of a different type (do you really want to spend more of your life on hold to helplines or making stilted pleas for support from chatbots?).

As a response to the problems of private solutions, it's common to call on governments to provide universal, comprehensive care systems. In fact, with barely an exception, every time I've discussed this book with friends, acquaintances and strangers, the immediate response has been that the government should provide more care services (with, presumably, a silent and unsaid 'so we don't have to' after their pronouncement). But can governments provide universal, comprehensive care systems that would meet our needs sufficiently? Yes and no. Of course, governments can use taxation revenues to fund wide-ranging and relatively comprehensive care services, like those Line experiences in Norway. It's complex, costly and never perfect – but it's doable, if political will exists. However, this doesn't remove the caregivers from their situation. In several of the stories we've witnessed in these pages, government services are present, and yet life still seems to be too hard for the caregivers involved. This truth undermines the implicit assumption when people invoke the idea of a 'national care service' or similar that it'll mean none of 'us' will have to care for our family members, or at most that we'll do so residually around more important things, like, presumably, work.

I sought in previous chapters to explain why this is never the case. Briefly rehearsing those crucial points, they were that first, the bodily reality of care means it is erratic, and public services require some degree of 'plannability'. We'd still need all the changes to the work world described in Chapter 7 in order to meet the unpredictable demands of care, regardless of the state provision.

Second, caregivers are needed to navigate, oversee and organise with the services provided. Kirsty Woodard, who created Ageing Without Children, explains it like this: 'It's the adult children who battle the care system for you to get the services . . . The people who talk to all the services, it's the children. They kind of oil the wheels that make it work. Otherwise, it's just lots of emails that don't get read . . . what happens if there isn't an adult child to do what's needed – what happens then?' Woodard is pointing out that our care system, as it's currently constituted, can't function without adult children playing a role. While she wants there to be advocates provided for those who are ageing without children, her point shows that providing government services doesn't remove the need for family and friends from the equation. At most, it reduces their involvement, but brief conversations with caregivers about navigating bureaucracies will quickly disabuse you of the idea that this is more than a minimal reduction.

Third, love exists. A substantial proportion of care is provided not because of the lack of an alternative, but because we love each other. Recently, I was speaking with a friend about this book and its likely contents. 'So, would you have wanted to care for your mum if there was a national care service available?' she asked. I answered that 'want' felt like the wrong verb. No part of me *wanted* to be in that circumstance. I can still barely bring myself to think about lengthy stretches of her illness. It's like my mind has large, dark curtains cloaking parts of it, corners that it refuses to observe, and that sometimes become upsettingly exposed as I try to sleep at night. I did not *want* to care for my mother, because I did not *want* any of it to be happening, at all, ever. But I did *need* to care for her. I didn't have a choice. Not just because of the social opprobrium my refusal would have provoked as her childless adult daughter. But because she was my mother. Imperfect and at times fractious as our relationship was, I felt as if there was a cord linking us that required me to do for her what I could. If more help had been available, I would gladly have taken it. But would I have wanted to be at work instead of coaxing her through physiotherapy exercises when she lost mobility for the third time after a hospital stint? Would I have wanted to be replying to emails instead of listening to her tell me about my great-aunt Coralie and that secret conversation she had with her? No. I'm far from alone in this feeling, based on my conversations with other caregivers. When I asked Tracy to describe caregiving in a few words, she said 'stressful' and 'emotionally draining', followed quickly by: 'But I'm thankful for the time that I have with my dad, and I wouldn't want anybody else doing it. I'm glad I can do it.'

Then there is the oft-overlooked issue of the preferences of those in need of care. Many people want loved ones to provide their care, or at least be nearby if someone else is washing and dressing them. Are we willing to decide as a society that we'll disregard the preferences of our most vulnerable? I hope not.

Finally, the idea that the government is a benign force isn't a universal truth. There are many groups of people for whom public provision would come with concerns that aren't present if care is provided by people whom they know. Eric and his husband Scott had paid care workers provided through Scott's health insurance, rather than by the government, but their case is a useful example of the worries that can arise with external sources of help, whether from government or market: 'I was like, 'Oh God, oh God, I hope it's somebody that's tolerant of two gay men here in an urban flat, going through this together.' LGBTQ communities, racialised people, undocumented migrants and sex industry workers may all have reasons to avoid paid care workers from government agencies entering their intimate spaces. In this way, having governments providing crucial support can block many in our societies from accessing that help. In the USA, Immigration and Customs Enforcement (ICE) has a 'sensitive locations' policy, barring it from making arrests at hospitals except in extraordinary circumstances. But there are grey areas. ICE is reported to have detained children needing emergency care and to have targeted undocumented people as they visit sick family members.[8] Research published in 2021 exploring the main barriers for undocumented people trying to access healthcare in Sweden found that 'fear of being taken by police/authorities' was prominent.[9] These are two very different countries, but in neither is government a friend to all.

The missing third option

There is a third option. It's hiding in many of the stories throughout the preceding pages, threads glinting within the familiar battle tapestries of private versus public. It's in Katy's assertion that 'you need networks of people you can rely on to do this bit or that bit . . . Probably it would have to be ten people who all did a tiny little bit of the whole.' It's in the small acts of support provided to each other by the women of OWCH, but also in their commitment to being outward-facing and part of their communities, 'not a coven'. It's in the COVID-19 mutual-aid groups that emerged, fungi-like, across our lands during our global health crisis. It's in the notion of kinning, a reimagined form of family that is porous and permeable, able to be creative with new relationships, constituted by the continual practice of responding to one another's needs. It's in the relationships that have been created among Cottam's Circle members, and between the women of my own small circle too.

These examples are thin but promising threads of a 'commons of care'. Most simply, a commons is a resource that nobody owns, but everyone can use. It could be a patch of land used to graze animals, or a river that's shared for washing or drinking. Lots of commons exist today, many more abstract than fields or rivers. Language is one. I don't own English; nor do you. Nor does the *Oxford English Dictionary* or the government. But we all use it and, furthermore, we all reshape it through our usage. There are lots of commons online too, such as open-source software repositories. There remains a surprising amount of land and other natural resources held in common in the world today, too, though we often don't realise it. This is partly due to the success of the 'tragedy of the commons' idea, famously expounded by American ecologist Garrett Hardin and later successfully refuted by Nobel Prize-winner Professor Elinor Ostrom. The 'things' themselves – land, water, language, software, etc. – alone don't constitute a commons, though. Without people using and collectively stewarding them, they're just a thing, an empty patch of forgotten land, a dead language. To have a commons, we need the thing that's held in common, but we need to be *commoning*, or acting in common, too. This means sharing responsibility collectively for that 'thing', and continually reproducing it by interacting with it and each other. A commons, then, is both the thing itself and the connected human activities that mean it's used *in common*.

On the journey in these pages so far, we've witnessed caregiving. Not the sanitised, Snow White version of patriarchal history, nor the commodified capitalist notion that treats it as a production line of tasks. Real care, rarely witnessed, desperately in need of recognition: Line living with no dreams; Ulla trying each day to be her husband's 'possibility maker'; Karen navigating her father's moods while observing her mother's decline; capable Ayesha finding herself broken and depressed; Eric tending to his memories of beloved Scott; Josie struggling valiantly to make ends meet; Katy getting screwed financially; Safa ignoring playground jibes about her sister; Carlyle and Barb working out new ways of living now that everything has changed; Tracy trying not to think about what's to come; and many more. We've refused to turn away from the concrete bodily reality of care, and have found that far from being a fluffy and nebulous concept, caregiving is constituted by a series of tangible actions and describable relationships. Instead of blades of grass on a plot of land, then, or a piece of software in the digital ether, our commons of care would be made up of these actions and relationships. It would make care a visible part of all our lives, not just those of people we now call 'caregivers', who happen to be mainly women and utterly exhausted under the isolating strain.

In their book *Free, Fair and Alive: The Insurgent Power of the Commons*, which explores the meaning of the commons and principles for making it a reality, experts David Bollier and Silke Helfrich write: 'The commons involves an identity shift. It requires that people evolve into different roles and perspectives. It demands new ways of relating to other people. It requires that we reassess who matters in our economy and society, and how essential work gets done.' It is, if you like, a combination of kinning – our reimagined, broader families – and our interdependent understandings of our 'selves' turned into practical actions and choices. As Bollier and Helfrich have also pointed out, defining granular specifics of the commons is unwise, because it's so inherently human that it will be very dependent on each context. This is something we struggle to understand in an era of mass production and mass services. It's a different conception of equality, shifting it from the ideal of 'the same provided to everyone' (which doesn't exist in reality), to one that instead seeks to ensure each has what they need. Nor is it transactional in a market sense, where each person calculates what they put in and expects to receive the same in return. Instead, it works based on that idea of 'general reciprocity' we encountered in Chapter 4: we give within our ability, and we receive when we need to, but with no 'amounts' or 'time frames' attached. Essentially, we each put energy into stitching our collective care net, and we each get to fall into it and be held by it when needed.

While Bollier and Helfrich are rightly wary of defining specifics, Deirdre's situation provides an obvious example of what could be different. One week, on our group support call in 2020, she explained that she'd only moved to the area in north-west England where she and her ailing husband live shortly before his rapid deterioration. She hadn't had time to establish strong social networks there before her life was thoroughly curtailed by care, adding to her isolation even before the COVID-19 pandemic.

It struck me as bizarre that when we move geographically, we move into a place with new transport links, and amenities like supermarkets or schools, but most of the time, we have no notion of exploring the social structures, and no concept of entering into a potential kinship network. There is no welcome from a mutual-aid society, no encouragement to join a circle, no process to initiate kinning. We unpack our things, arrange our furniture, and exist isolated as if on an island. Our streets have Neighbourhood Watches to look out for burglars, but no comparable structures of caring. I have heard of places where things are done differently – a neighbourhood in Sheffield with its own local group, a market town in mid-Wales – but they're exceptions to the miserable rule. And it's not as if there wouldn't be people in Deirdre's community with whom she could build support and kinship. Statistically, it's highly likely there are others in the vicinity who are isolated, lonely and struggling. A commons of care changes that, without falling into the pitfalls of government-provided services, and while being intimately linked to the local area in which it's situated. It also confronts us with our own role in caregiving, unlike the idea of 'infrastructure', which is usually taken to mean something outside of ourselves and provided *for* us, not *by* us. It is the bold and hopeful solution we've been searching for.

But we must be clear about what this vision is not. In 2010, the UK voted in a new government in the form of a coalition between the Conservative Party and the Liberal Democrat Party. The flagship policy of the former's election manifesto was called the Big Society. 'A country is at its best when the bonds between people are strong,' wrote Conservative Party leader and future Prime Minister David Cameron in the preface. The Big Society would be a new approach, apparently, one focused on 'social responsibility' and not 'big government'. It promised to redistribute power from the central state to individuals, families and local communities. It was time for everyone to play their part. Except they were expected to play that part for free, with no real power, rights or entitlements, and without any changes to the material resources, injustices or wage labour that shaped their lives. In reality, the Big Society appeared to be an exhortation to volunteer more in local communities while the government cut vital services. Cameron and his Big Society were like those infomercials you flick on to by accident: a too-good-to-be-true new product, presented with a smarmy smile and slick words covering its flimsy materials and construction. The problem wasn't with the idea that people might hold solutions. It was the cynical deployment of that idea to avoid governmental responsibility for people's needs, without ceding any power or resources, or addressing deep inequalities.

Around the world, there's been growing interest in an allied approach to the Big Society that focuses on coaching people into self-support. These 'asset-based' approaches are explicitly aimed at reducing people's need for, and use of, government-provided services. 'Help build capacity and self-sufficiency instead of "providing services"', reads one report promoting this type of model.[10] Lucy's story is recounted as an example of success. Lucy had depression, anxiety and a learning disability. This made it hard for her to work, and so she'd received sickness support from the government. However, her benefits were stopped after she was assessed as fit for work by an inaccurate government assessment. With the help of the 'local area coordinator', a kind of coach deployed by some asset-based approaches, Lucy was able to challenge the decision and get her benefits reinstated. This was great news for Lucy, but it also obscures some rather important facts.

In the UK, where Lucy lived, badly run 'work capability

assessments' have repeatedly certified people fit for work who are patently not, including the terminally ill. In fact, thousands have died only shortly after being designated fit for work, so severe were their health issues.[11] Lucy is just one of many thousands of people affected. While an asset-based model worked well in her case, it's premised on an individualistic approach that sidesteps the deep and unjust flaws in the system itself. In its determination to ask 'the right questions – instead of focusing on deficits', and to help 'people focus on their own vision for a good life',[12] this model obscures the fact that deficits are real and sometimes beyond a person's control. What good is it to ask someone about their vision for the good life if their pay is so low they're choosing between heating and eating? How moral is it to ask someone to identify their 'assets' if they're living in damp housing with their disabled child, who is contracting infections because of the mould? Is it acceptable to have a solution that only helps one mother in that situation, instead of going to the government and demanding change? Is it logical to promote a solution that focuses on individuals, rather than asking what better ways we might organise our lives? Arguably, Cottam's Circle could be understood as falling foul of the same issues, although its method of combining people together holds a political potential missing when an approach is solely between a 'professional' and the person whom they're 'helping to help themselves'. Regardless, there must be a role for us, the people, as caregivers or soon-to-be-caregivers, as old or pre-old, disabled or pre-disabled, *and* a role for government too, addressing these large-scale deficits and injustices.

The role of government

There's a dual role for governments to play if we're to solve the crisis of care. First, accepting that we're very far away from having the kinds of resources and relationships that would constitute a commons of care, and that some diseases are more advanced than relatively untrained people can support, we need to maintain a standard of state-provided services. It's not realistic or safe to expect a commoning approach to provide direct care to people in advanced stages of dementia, for example. Likewise, delivering food to someone's address is one thing, but changing a feeding tube is entirely another. And there will always be some people who lack kin or whose loved ones are also struggling with health issues. For these reasons and more, we need governments to provide care services, and these include services to caregivers themselves, like respite so that they can take a break. Increasing the number of care jobs available will also be common sense for the economy in the future, as the climate crisis pressures workers to leave high-carbon industries and move into cleaner sectors. There's much important experimentation with business models going on around the world, with interesting projects creating arrangements that are more effective and humane than current privatised services, such as cooperative models funded by government. These need to be built into government provisioning, and the profit focus removed. Others have written extensively about these aspects; our interest here is how, with that in place, the government can play a role in the commons of care. Hilary Cottam described her vision, exemplified in Circle, as a model of abundance – the more people got involved, the more resources there were. Well, the role of government that we'll explore now is the precondition of that abundance, of a commons of care. Ideas like the Big Society don't understand this. They give us *permission* to relate to each other more deeply and effectively, but no real *power*. It's like handing someone a driver's licence but banning them from buying a car.

We need rights and recognition

First, we need the legal right to provide care for our loved ones. In the previous chapter, we saw how important this is within the work world. Much of the language supporting Biden's plans and comparable UK campaigns has focused on how providing more paid care support services will free people up to remain in their jobs. Waged work is our priority; love is demoted. We can't reimagine families or build a commons of care without more time to do so, and that means we need a legally enshrined right to provide care. This will rebalance the scales between work and care, opening up time and energy for the important 'species activities' of both kinning and commoning. Making it a universal right, rather than one only relating to the workplace, is important, too, because it will be applicable to other kinds of scenarios that currently prevent us from providing care to loved ones. Recall the attempted deportation of Ms Inferrera in Chapter 4. A universal human right to provide care could prevent future cases like this from occurring. We do have a right to family life already under the UN Universal Declaration of Human Rights, but this is understood as the traditional family, which does little to help a future in which that notion is so archaic.

Having a right to provide care for loved ones, and the changes flowing from that, would immediately make caregivers visible. This would have huge benefits for caregivers' mental health. Ample evidence shows how important it is for people's wellbeing that they feel recognised for the value they bring. How can we recognise what doesn't appear to exist?

When I asked Josie what word she'd use to describe caregiving, she barely paused before she said, 'Nightmare.' Then she thought for a moment and continued: 'There's the nice aspects, where it's nice to be needed and to feel like you're doing a really important job. I think that's the thing, really. You feel that about yourself, and then the system lets you down, because they make you feel like you're not important and you're not doing anything special.' A right to care could change this, along with the suggestions provided in Chapter 5 about our collective education. We'd all know what caregiving is, that it matters enough to have rights attached, and that it should be respected as something both valiant and normal, arduous and loving.

We need money

'Love is not enough; care requires material resources,' writes Professor Nakano Glenn in *Forced to Care*. Providing rights and recognition for caregivers is important, but risks beckoning us down an undesirable path back towards the angel in the house, where women are valorised but left worse off because of care. We live in a world that makes money a necessity for survival. And yet, we are creatures who can't work for portions of our lives, either because we're impaired ourselves or because we're tending to someone else. These two facts together mean we need a caregiver's income. This can be done in various ways, and it's beyond the scope of this book to explore them in depth. Suffice to say, the process of determining a caregiver's income should start by listening to caregivers about their costs and needs, before going on to design a solution based on their experiences.

In some countries and states, caregivers can be formally employed to support a loved one, with either the government paying the salary directly to the caregiver, or the person receiving the care paying them out of entitlements they receive from government or private health insurance. This seems to be well liked where it does exist and deserves further exploration. Tracy was paid by her mother's health insurance to care for her because she was already a qualified medical assistant. But when it was time to give up her job and care for her father, the insurance company turned around and said, 'We never should have reimbursed you, because you're a family member.' She tells me how infuriating it is to know her parents paid into their scheme for fifty-odd years, but a loophole has been used to avoid paying out. 'It's frustrating because they'll pay a complete stranger to come in and take care of my dad, someone he doesn't know, but they aren't going to reimburse a family member that would probably give better care, in my opinion. It just doesn't make sense.'

It's the old Snow White trap, the one that thinks it's laudable that Tracy wants to care lovingly for her father, but apparently also thinks she doesn't need to eat or pay bills to do so. Insurance companies must pay income to family members who provide care when they ask for it. And both they and governments, depending on which is applicable in the context, need to make direct payments to people while they're on caregivers' leave from jobs, or top up their income if they've had to reduce their days but not leave entirely.

Clearly, a sensible caregiver's income needs to be set at a liveable rate. Katy was a secondary school teacher before she left to be her husband's caregiver. In the UK, a teacher who'd been teaching for several years at that level might earn around £35,000. This translates to around £528 a week in pay, after taxes: markedly more than the £67.60 she gets today.

'I think when you don't have a salary of your own anymore, and that's what somebody says you're worth, that has a big knock-on effect on your confidence, knowing that you're not worth ten pounds a day when you're doing so much,' she tells me.

Caregivers' income could be pinned to someone's pre-care income, providing Katy with respectful remuneration. However, income-replacement schemes that are pinned to prior earnings do nothing to address pre-existing disparities along gender, race and other lines. A justice-based approach could include a sliding scale of income replacement, with a higher percentage of income paid to those who earned less before care, and a lower percentage to those who earned more. This is, in fact, what Biden proposed for his new caregiver's leave, as we saw earlier. Whatever the arrangement, caregivers' income needs to be understood not as an *allowance* but as an *entitlement*. The difference is important. The former implies you're lucky to be in receipt of it, the latter that receiving it is your right.

As we saw in Chapter 1, it isn't only the present financial well-being of caregivers that takes a hit under current arrangements. Their future solvency is also harmed, because being unable to work, or having to work less, reduces savings and social security entitlements. It's necessary, then, that caregivers receive social security credits for the duration of time that their working lives are affected by care. If we manage to move away from the idea that caregiving is something only 'some' people do, and that those people are 'other', i.e. not you, and instead move toward the provider-caregiver model described in Chapter 7, it becomes obvious that this is necessary, because otherwise everyone's old age income will be markedly reduced. Are we intending everyone to live the elderly portions of their lives in penury?

There's a paradox at work here: politicians understand – or at least pay lip service to – the need to fund free care services better. This pays people to care for strangers. But when it comes to kin caregivers, the idea of paying them seems novel and unlikely, even though they're actually there in the first place. And we do have the money – it's just spent on other things, like the astronomical sums spent on weaponry we hope never to use, or on 'incentives' for corporations to build new facilities and create more (precarious, underpaid) jobs, and so on. We can find the money for caregivers – if we choose to do so. In 2018, a new US law came into force called the RAISE Family Caregivers Act, the acronym standing for Recognise, Assist, Include, Support and Engage. It established an advisory council on caregivers and required the Secretary of Health and Human Services to develop a national family caregiving strategy. Subsequently, in September 2021, the advisory council published its first report.[13] It recognises that caregivers face financial hardship, and includes a recommendation to 'decrease the negative financial impacts for family caregivers on both a short- and long-term basis'.[14] However, it fails to recommend an income for kin caregivers, instead focusing on making the cost of paid care services cheaper. While this is better than nothing, it falls into the trap of thinking that more services will mean kin don't have to perform any care – which, as we've seen, is incorrect.

We need power and autonomy

With rights, recognition and money, caregivers would already be far better off than they are currently. But they could still be lonely islands, merely better paid and with time off work. To join our islands, we need legal changes and resources that enable us to create our commons of care.

In 2018 in Canada, the New Leaf Project gave one-off lump sums of CAN $7,500 to fifty people who'd recently become homeless. They were entirely free to choose how they spent the money. Researchers followed them, along with a second group who didn't get any money, over the next year and a half to see how the two groups fared. It turned out that if people were given the money they needed, and autonomy in their decisions about how to spend it, they could do just fine. The people in the first group found stable housing more quickly than the other group, and spent money on food, clothing and rent, while their expenditure on alcohol, cigarettes and drugs reduced.[15] The results have been described as 'beautifully surprising' by the CEO of one of the organisations involved, although they needn't have been. Similarly successful experiments have been carried out previously, including one twenty years prior, also in Canada, in which a doctor began 'prescribing' money to his homeless patients, many of whom then found secure housing within a year or less.

The point is, when people are given money (which, in today's world, is often synonymous with power) and the right to use that money as best suits their needs, things can work out rather well. But today, our political systems are set up to protect their own functioning more than they are to respond to our participation and demands. Bollier and Helfrich recount an example of the problem we face: 'In Bologna, Italy, an elderly woman wanted a simple bench in the neighbourhood's favourite gathering spot. When residents asked the city government if they could install a bench themselves, a perplexed city bureaucracy replied that there were no procedures for doing so.'[16] Bologna, along with many other cities around the world, including Barcelona, Ghent and Turin, have since sought to change this, introducing new regulations focused on enabling commoning to occur.

Commoning requires these changes, including alterations to legal powers and money to go with them. Buildings need to be bought and furnished; utilities, transport and food need to be paid for. Some models may also wish to pay members for specific roles. Local communities should be given substantial sums of money with which to build these new structures and maintain them. This is a strange hybrid of politics, but a necessary one for the era in which we find ourselves, and one that will transition to something more purely 'commons-based' in time. Helfrich has explained that 'there can be contributions to a commons without commoning. This is where the state comes in. The state can contribute to commons without necessarily participating in commoning. It should also secure the rights of all citizens, not just the rights of commoners, and support constructive relations among commons.'[17]

This could be misunderstood as a kind of charitable stance from government: 'handing out' money to the people, a Robin Hood in bureaucratic form. But for us to avoid the pitfalls of the Big Society and comparable political projects, we need to step away from models where government keeps most of the power while giving out small portions to tide us over. Instead, government must be like a light bulb – something that draws in and then emits power, not keeping it for itself but enabling that which is around it. Happily, this is also an image that connotes the wisdom of new and exciting ideas. The light bulb approach means a substantial handover of assets, like community buildings, cash, and most crucially, the power to make decisions about how those things are used. 'It is one thing to organise communally the way we want to eat,' wrote political theorist and activist of the commons idea, Silvia Federici, '. . . and then ask the State to pay for it, and it is the opposite thing to ask the State to organise our meals.'[18]

The state is a useful apparatus for drawing in energy – in the form of money via taxation – but we need it to transfer that energy to us so that we can organise our communities effectively. This would open the door to whole new ways of organising care, from funding self-organised teams of neighbourhood advocates to support those who are ageing without children, to running community centres where caregivers can find solidarity and advice. Importantly, those new options would be defined and designed by the people using them. Perhaps, like Hilary Cottam's Circle, some local areas would start membership groups for care and community, while others would come up with completely new ways of supporting each other, too.

Without that transfer, we risk finding ourselves with all the responsibility and none of the power. This is the nature of 'volunteering' under models like the Big Society and much of what passes for community involvement in social projects today. When Silke Helfrich died hiking in the Liechtenstein Alps in November 2021, she left behind her a wealth of urgent, practical work on the idea of the commons. For her, the distinction between volunteering versus having real power to organise as a community was clear:

> The terms volunteering and self-organisation relate to one another like 'parliamentarians' to 'democracy' or 'parents' to 'family'. Self-organisation describes a mode of organisation . . . that can take various forms. Voluntary work, on the other hand, has a role within an existing order.[19]

And, as we've seen, the existing order isn't working. Taking on a role within it will mean we have more to do, but without the power, money and time to do it. It will mean being told by government to be grateful for paltry hand-outs while it continues to gatekeep public services in attempts to keep costs down, so that money can be spent elsewhere, on things that we have not said are our priorities. It will mean thousands more stories like Lucy's and Deirdre's. In the commons of care, we aren't 'volunteering'; we're acting both for each other and ourselves, continually creating a web of care that holds us all as we travel through life.

We need care-full spaces

'Trying to create co-housing creates challenges with planning departments,' Bruno Friedel tells me. In the spirit of government both getting out of the way of the commons of care and creating the fertile soil in which it can grow, I've asked him what obstacles exist for co-housing, given that it's such an obvious way of kinning, an important node in the commons. His examples show acutely how far we've come from living in common with each other:

> In Leeds in the north of the UK, a co-housing community . . . wanted to have 0.5 car parking spaces per household and that was a curve ball for the local planning department. They have expectations that there should be one car per household, so nothing is set up to cope with a shared approach. And in some countries, trying to have a common house – a central shared space – can cause problems because the authorities don't know how to categorise it. It's not residential or commercial.

Isn't that ridiculous? What's happened to us? Commoning is practical work involving lots of energy, time and responsibility, not nice words about friendships and love. When there are obstacles like these every few metres, people lose energy for this project.

In another example of how our building practices ignore the nature of human life, many homes can't accommodate people with limited mobility. Can yours? I bet it can't, unless someone like Katy has lived there before you. When I ask how her living situation has affected her caring responsibilities, she tells me:

> We knew [my husband] wouldn't be able to climb stairs soon, so we had our garage converted and an extension to make into a downstairs bedroom and a wet room. It was a nightmare getting planning permission, but we were able to do [it] so that before he could no longer get up the stairs, which are very steep, old, cottage-style stairs, we had that in place. We're probably at a point now where we need some more grab rails and things like that. So we're on our second iteration of making some changes. And we made sure that when the bedroom was built, it had joists strong enough for hoists for when that's necessary [for lifting him], and the shower has push buttons that are designed to be easy for him.

They were only able to make these changes because Katy's uncle died, and so she had some money. Although there are grants available for people to make home modifications due to disabilities, she tells me that 'people with MND [motor neurone disease] often die before the approval comes through'. She says she can't imagine how someone would cope if they were renting and so couldn't make the necessary changes. For Carlyle and Barb, that was the case, so they had to move. It's a curious thing, that we build dwellings only functional for a slim portion of our lives. The omission of truly accessible, disability-friendly aspects from home-building is a symptom of our deeper attempt to forget that such things can and will happen. If we understood ourselves not as 'able', but rather as temporarily able, or, if you like, 'pre-disabled', how would we build then?

In the introduction to their lauded 1984 book *Making Space,* the Matrix Feminist Design Co-operative wrote that 'Buildings do not control our lives' but they do 'reflect the dominant values in our society'. Along with a failure to fathom spaces that can accommodate sharedness and impairments, we lack spaces that are explicitly for care but aren't ostracising for those who use them. As we've seen, some of the problems faced by caregivers are that they lack breaks from providing care, are isolated, and that the person for whom they care doesn't want to go to special day centres nor be cared for by strangers. One solution to this could be the creation of 'care cafés', community centres that support and service care needs, but in a broad-ranging and attractive way.

Julian Siravo is Urban Research Lead for UK-based think-tank Autonomy. He focuses on how architecture and spatial design can be used to achieve societal goals. He's proposed creating centres in communities that provide leisure, support and activities for people who need care and those who care for them, whether they're kin caregivers or paid care workers. A small paid staff would be on site, probably becoming familiar over time to the people attending the centre, and so enabling the rapport-building that's crucial to care (and to giving kin caregivers breaks). Designing these spaces well, from the sofas to the signage, he explains, is crucial when it comes to getting people to use them. 'Most people do not want to identify with being old, or ill, or in need of care,' he tells me. 'But when we frame a space as a space where you go for certain activities, rather than as a space where you go because you are a certain person, that makes all the difference.' He envisions these centres – or cafés, as I prefer to conceive them, due to the word's more welcoming, less pathologising connotation – as including a range of professional services that are useful to the people who attend, such as advisors on government entitlements and medical professionals. That aspect is vital for success; no one – not caregivers, not those receiving care – will want to go somewhere that designates them lacking in some way or that fails to recognise and respect their three-dimensional selves.

Siravo's idea is allied with the work of both Hilary Cottam and Carers Worldwide. Cottam's Circle is effectively creating a care café, except without the singular bricks-and-mortar presence – rather, her approach is dispersed throughout a neighbourhood, manifesting in the practical actions its members take. Carers Worldwide has promoted the creation of twenty-five community caring centres in India, Nepal and Bangladesh. Although part of their rationale is to enable kin caregivers to leave their loved one while they earn money, the centres also provide services that support caregivers directly, including counselling. In an allied intervention, Carers Worldwide has initiated the creation of peer-support groups, which have now begun creating pooled savings, much like a friendly society of the past. 'They've saved nearly £70,000 . . . to use in emergency situations. or if one of them needs to set up an income stream, like a small kiosk,' executive director Anil Patil tells me. In addition, grants are provided to carers in the form of loans via a revolving fund; once they begin to earn an income, they repay the loan to the carers' group at a low rate of interest, and the money is then available to be used by another carer.

Speaking with Siravo and Patil about these concepts, my mind is flooded with stories of caregivers, including my own, and all the small ways in which this could have helped us. The idea of having a special space – an entire floor, in Siravo's design – dedicated to our support and respite is compelling and almost tear-inducing. When my mum got sick, I was on medication for depression. This has been a long-standing element of my mental world, and the medication I take has been very effective. I could only get one month's worth prescribed at a time, however, meaning that each month, I had to go to the doctor's and post a slip of paper in the 'repeat prescription' box, then return forty-eight hours or more later to collect my new script. Shuttling between work, which was around forty-five minutes from where I lived, and my mum's house or hospital, combined with my overwhelming exhaustion, made it impossible to remember and schedule these twice-monthly trips. I just about managed for a handful of months, and then I gave up. I stopped the medication abruptly without tapering off, against medical advice. With the right set-up and powers, a centre like the one Siravo describes could have changed this, and perhaps that break-up that occurred several months later wouldn't have led me to such a dark place.

Training for caregivers could also be offered at these sites. 'Informal' caregivers are performing all sorts of tasks at home that you might think would only be done by a nurse: administering injections and medication, cleaning wounds and food tubes, changing diapers, operating dialysis machines, and so on. Many of these tasks need some degree of training before they can be done safely. The small number of training courses that already exist in the world have had good results. A programme pioneered by the Dana-Farber Cancer Institute and Boston Children's Hospital trains caregivers for several days before a central line (a catheter going into a large vein) is inserted, and a nurse is also sent to the home to support family caregivers. This programme has 'dramatically reduced bloodstream infections stemming from care at home'.

Siravo thinks this sort of porosity between formal sites of care, like hospitals, and informal ones, like the home, is crucial to constructing a commons of care. 'These spaces were really conceived to mix the accountability and professionalism of a space like a hospital, with the more intimate and caring qualities of a family environment.' This is important not just for the support and flexibility it can offer caregivers, but also because it undoes some of the segregation of bodily care. 'We usually think of buildings as containers of activity,' he continues. 'We often overlook the way that they represent a signal to the city. I think how much we celebrate and acknowledge an activity is expressed in the position that we give that activity, and the visibility we give it in the urban fabric.' Buildings, then, become part of recognising caregivers and care in our society, normalising neediness. They become a crucial element of the commons, just like the rights and entitlements we also need.

And what about the spaces between dwellings? Many urban planners and architects have been advocating for designs that better reflect human activities and needs. The New Urbanist movement cohered in the 1990s and states that: 'New Urbanism is a movement united around the belief that our physical environment has a direct impact on our chances for happy, prosperous lives.' Members promote principles such as 'liveable' streets that can be walked around easily, the importance of shops and schools that are accessible without private vehicles, and planning shaped around 'universally accessible public spaces and community institutions'. This is the bricks and mortar, the concrete and cement, of caregiving. Because if we don't pass each other in our daily lives, if we don't stand in line at the same small shop, or nod hello as we go to post a letter, or see that same guy down the street washing his car with his kid every Saturday, or know what time the old lady at number twelve usually goes for her daily constitutional . . . if we don't observe, notice and exist in a web of these small human activities, then we don't know each other. And if we don't know each other, we don't care.

Jane Jacobs opened her iconic 1961 book *The Death and Life of Great American Cities* as she meant to go on: 'This book is an attack on current city planning and rebuilding.' In her subsequent tirade against the ills of urban America, she highlights the importance of having streets that are used by people in all those small everyday ways. One day, she watched from her window as a 'suppressed struggle' between a man and a young girl of around eight years old took place in the street below. She thought that 'the man seemed to be trying to get the girl to go with him'. Jacobs considered intervening, but then saw a woman emerge from the butcher's shop nearby, arms folded, eyeing the man. The delicatessen owner emerged, too, and two men from a bar, then the locksmith, the 'fruit man' and the owner of the laundry. All stood and watched. 'The man did not know it,' she writes, 'but he was surrounded . . . nobody was going to allow a little girl to be dragged off.' Thankfully, it turned out to be a father and daughter, nothing more sinister. While Jacobs focuses largely on how lively and walkable streets improve people's safety, the same can also be said for improving people's care and the support of their caregivers.

Much of what I've said above could be misunderstood as being relevant 'only' for people with impairments. But every time a decision is made that makes it harder to live somewhere with a disability – harder to wheel a wheelchair along, to know there's a safe, calm, outdoor space somewhere close to your home, or to be within a few short minutes' walking distance of a food shop, and so on that decision adds to the secret tally of suffering of the care-giver. I have too many examples of this to enumerate. Here's one.

In early 2018, a handful of months after her cancer diagnosis, my mother nearly died from the allergic reaction to medication I've already described. Back at home after a long stint in hospital, she was physically weak and afraid of trying to go out in case she couldn't walk far enough to get back home. There was a shop around four minutes' walk from her house, and it became our goal to get her there – the park, about seven minutes' walk, would be the next goal after that. Nothing bad happened, except that I have a scene scored into my heart that sometimes plays on repeat, unbidden. Every day, with the odd skipped one if she felt too bad, we tried to go out of her front door. A few steps, her arm resting in the crook of mine, ignoring people rubbernecking at us as they passed. We got to the corner of her street on the second day, about two metres from her front door. It took us two or three weeks to get her strong enough to walk to that shop and back. Consistent, loving practice, encouragement, cajoling, respectful pulling back . . . the caregiver's tasks are more than a crooked arm.

Finally, she was ready to try alone. And that's the image I have of her in my mind. Playing repeatedly. Her form, several metres along the pavement, so much smaller than it used to be, her upper arms glued to her sides as if she was trying to form a shell around her body, her forearms at right angles, ready to protect her from the strange, fearful world into which she had been regurgitated. A scared bird. I felt like I think mothers must when watching their child do something that could hurt them. All of me lurched inside. I wanted to run away and hold her at the same time. The reversal of our roles, the up-ending of our lives, the brittle exhaustion now permeating every waking hour, how fragile she looked out there on the suburban street, which suddenly seemed to be a jungle of dangers. She picked her way slowly and gingerly around poorly laid paving stones, and then she was out of sight, around a corner. She didn't fall. She didn't get run over. Nothing bad happened at all. But those ten minutes of my life burn in me. That is what being a caregiver means.

Could we please make it a little easier?

The seeds of a new world

Too often, when governments are thought about in relation to care, people consider only the most obvious functions, conjuring visions of armies of care workers. These visions keep care firmly in its place – a thing done by other people, a thing that can be neatly circumscribed in our politics, thoughts and lives. This isn't how caregiving really works. Instead, it's everywhere, all the time. In people's homes, in their communities, on the streets and in workplaces. It permeates our world, both concretely and emotionally. We are living in a relatively new world in terms of life expectancy, family sizes and chronic diseases. We need a new model of care for that new world.

For political theorist and activist Silvia Federici, the seeds of this new world are to be planted in this very practice of commoning: 'the cooperation that we can develop among ourselves, which is most tested when confronted with the task of ensuring that the lives of those who are tied to wheelchairs or hospital beds do not become a living torture, as it is so often the case in our society'.[20] To grow these seeds will require us to overcome discomfort with very different ways of meeting our needs. It will require trust and confidence in ourselves and each other. It will require us to know that human relations are messy, and so commoning will be messy too, never final and never neatly solved. But, in case you hadn't noticed, both sides of the private/ public battle are messy too, wreaking havoc in caregivers' lives and, sometimes, killing people in the process. We'd need new skills to build our commons of care, skills for building relationships, knowing our boundaries, making decisions together, and holding people accountable for the prejudices they will inevitably bring to common spaces. All these things take time and learning, though happily there is already a wealth of education and experimentation that can point us in the right directions.

By following this path, we can inhabit a future in which someone visiting our world is as bemused as *Herland*'s Vandyck Jennings by our seeming lack of 'care'. Why is no one crying as they shuttle frantically between work and sick kin? Why is no one impoverished because someone they love is impaired? Why are there no harried women taking buses to strangers' houses to provide speedy bed baths and then do it all again to another stranger? Why is no one sitting lonely beside their mute loved one, wondering how the hell to survive another dawn? Because care would be everywhere, and it would be like asking a bird to interrogate the sky.

Conclusion

'. . . we are all fated to lose our carefully constructed sense of self, our physical strength, our health, our precious dignity and finally our lives. A refusal to tolerate this reality is a refusal to tolerate life . . .'

Mary Gaitskill[1]

There is a substantial obstacle in our path to this better future. The COVID-19 pandemic shocked people on many levels, not least the sudden proximity to death. Might that person coughing on the train have coronavirus? Will I touch a door handle that has this terrifying new germ on it? Should I be stockpiling food, buying oxygen tanks? In normal times, we live inside a denial of death. We can see the imprints of it all around us – homes designed for the fully able, nested in cities that actively disable people who function differently, the sole startling occasion that you saw someone in the street with an oxygen mask or a chemo scalp. We can't have life without death, and yet we have created life without death's presence.

In fact, some people want to eradicate death altogether. Maverick scientist Aubrey de Grey has spent decades spearheading research that he claims will one day end ageing. Arizona-based not-for-profit Alcor will take tens of thousands of dollars from you in return for freezing your corpse – the full body, or just the head if money's tight. At the time of writing, they have 184 'patients' stored in vacuum-insulated containers at subfreezing temperatures.[2] 'The patient,' says the website, 'will remain in long-term care until revival becomes possible.'

While wealthy people freeze their heads in the hope of Christ-like resurrections, the rest of us must face the truth about being human – that we are alive and we will die. Our bodies remind us of this daily by requiring us to nourish them and care for them, often through frequent bouts of sickness. Charles Darwin wrote:

> Man, with all his noble qualities, with sympathy which feels for the most debased, with benevolence which extends not only to other men but to the humblest living creature, with his god-like intellect which has penetrated into the movements and constitution of the solar system – with all these exalted powers – Man still bears in his bodily frame the indelible stamp of his lowly origin.[3]

The cultural anthropologist Ernest Becker put it rather more bluntly in his 1973 Pulitzer Prize-winning book, *The Denial of Death*: 'We are gods with anuses.' Darwin and Becker sought to articulate the dissonance at the core of being human – that is, of being a self-conscious being. We have the same biological urge as other organisms to avoid death, yet we also know that our death is inevitable. Thus, we seek refuge in the worlds we create around us. The meanings with which we imbue them keep at bay the inescapable fact of our creatureliness, with its ignominious mortality and defecation. As Becker once explained: 'We build character and culture in order to shield ourselves from the devastating awareness of our underlying helplessness and the terror of our inevitable death.'[4]

Scholars who took forward Becker's work and turned it into a formal theory (called 'terror-management theory') have since amassed a rich body of experimental evidence that shows fear of death appears to have a profound effect on our thoughts, feelings and behaviours. They've shown that we need to feel we're valuable participants in a meaningful universe in order to cope with this fear.[5] I think this holds the key to solving the 'care crisis' in a deeper and more fundamental way than changes in government chambers or local neighbourhoods. The real care crisis is within and between each of us, because together we create a society that sidesteps the brute truth about human frailty, and therefore fails to create the systems and structures we need.

How can we feel meaningful if our lives are subsumed by care, but we live in a culture that doesn't respect care, or even want to acknowledge its existence? In which systems fail to provide for us and individuals recoil? In which our very homes can't accommodate its reality? How can we begin kinning with each other if we can't even cope with the idea that care is needed? It's no wonder caregivers are breaking down. For those who have been, or are, caregivers, the experiences and observations in these pages are intimately familiar. But if you're reading this and haven't been a caregiver, I have a message for you. We need you to be brave. You, in fact, need yourself to be brave, too, because care is in your future. You have a choice. You can adhere to the worldview that keeps sickness, injury and death at bay, that believes it to be 'unfair' when mortality strikes, as if there is a scale of justice somewhere that has been wrongly weighted, instead of merely chaos. You can rush full-speed at profit and status, erase wrinkles and surround yourself with the material accolades of a life lived in line with the values of advanced capitalism. Perhaps you can join Jeff Bezos on a giant phallus going into space, or sign up to have your head frozen. Above all, you can deny the fact that nothing you do will stave off death. In doing so, you can continue to stigmatise and ostracise caregivers, to make their lives even harder every single day.

Or you can be brave.

Make death part of your worldview, rather than something you use your worldview to keep at bay. Make it so that your sense of value rests in part on your ability to walk hand-in-hand with the knowledge of mortality, and, in so doing, hand-in-hand with the overlooked people on its frontline, the caregivers. We need you to be brave. If altruism isn't your thing, be brave because without this collective shift, you'll be the one broken.

'Really grasp that being mortal, while terrifying, can also make our lives sublime by infusing us with courage, compassion and concern for future generations.'[6] This is what the three psychologists who've worked on terror-management theory say towards the end of their book on the subject, *The Worm at the*

Core: On the Role of Death in Life. I'm not sure that mortality makes our lives sublime. Maybe it does. Maybe it also brings a lot of diaper-changing and the banal tragedies of loss. It doesn't really matter which is true though, or if both are, because, well, we *are* mortal. As Vladimir Nabokov wrote in *Speak, Memory*: 'The cradle rocks above an abyss, and common sense tells us that our existence is but a brief crack of light between two eternities of darkness.' We might as well get used to it. For me, this re-education about mortality has been the greatest lesson and the most brutal gift of being a caregiver.

In the pages of this book, we've done precisely what our fear-bound society fails to do: we've given our attention to caregivers. Their stories, and my own, are acts of courage and perseverance. The retelling of them was painful, cathartic, and necessary for each of us. We're grateful that you've paid us the respect of witnessing our experiences, not as animals glad for scraps, but because respect is the seed of a better future.

We stand on the brink of two futures. In one, care needs escalate and intensify, as we know they will. We stay faithful to our emaciated idea of the family, only realising when it's too late that this structure we thought was our safety net is instead a cage. We continue to work in the way we do now. We break our minds, bodies, social lives and relationships trying to meet the morality of the 'work ethic' while simultaneously tending to sick or impaired loved ones. We believe that care is a separable economic sector from our lives, a form of work that someone else should carry out on our behalf. We have a vague idea that this 'someone else' will be an impoverished migrant or a woman of colour, or perhaps, if we're inclined to such things, a lump of plastics and metals shaped to look like a sci-fi wet dream. We work, we care, we stumble and realise we're breaking, so, like several of us in these pages, we leave our jobs to be full-time caregivers. In the world as it is, without new rights and incomes, this cripples our financial security and, indeed, our very sense of identity. Our breaks come in the form of the weary hands of paid care workers, as underpaid as us, as rights-deprived as us, but lacking even the valorisation from which we can sometimes suckle a drop of comfort. Their children and elderly parents are left needful at home in poorer countries. Voids of care pock-mark the atlas so that richer countries can keep their pretence going, that crucial self-delusion, that we are gods and entropy is something best kept behind closed doors. In our own infirmity, when it comes, we sit alone in a room, but are told we're not alone, because a machine is talking to us. We repeat mantras of gratitude for the bounties of technology, trying to believe them as our skin hungers for human touch.

In the alternative future, some things remain the same. Care needs still escalate and intensify. Care remains hard, because love is hard. Care stays unpleasant at times, because bodies are unpleasant at times. And every person who walks through that hardship and unpleasantness, confronting the brutal facts of mortality, wrestling with the grief that comes stuck to the innards of love, is walking with their arms interlinked with others. They are held by the flexible, strong net of the commons, kept going each day by their voluptuous kinship practices, able to pause their work without racing into poverty or being judged as purposeless, safe in the knowledge that they have the right to do this very important thing, and that their life won't be stymied because of it. They live in homes and neighbourhoods with courageous architecture and planning, the kind that doesn't recoil in the face of our neediness, but builds it into the shapes of our lives so that we can be both needy and capable. They have been told since childhood that a time like this would come, so they expected it. Their pride isn't staked on being superior to providing care, attempting to jettison it to some 'other', whether a female relative, a poorer human or a machine. Rather, their confidence is that of those who have confronted the hardest parts of being human and kept their heart beating through it all.

Our best guides in reaching that second future are the caregivers themselves. They are experts by experience. In the spirit of which, let's conclude with the guidance of their own words. The caregivers I interviewed shared with me three things: what they missed from before they were caring, what they needed, and what they'd learned. I considered the same triad from my own experience. We present them to you, these things that you'll miss, need and learn as a caregiver. Turn to the next page, take in our words, linger over them, give them the respect of your attention, in the hope that if we can attend now to these messages, we can make the future better, for ourselves and all who come next.

Who Cares

What you'll miss

sleep

having a social life

naivety

the person your loved one used to be

sleep

going on holiday

feeling part of the world

being able to turn off your phone

sleep

the way you thought life would be

choice

belief in medicine working

292

sleep

the before of everything

dreams

illusions of freedom

sleep

shitting regularly

life being wide open

taking your loved one for granted

sleep

love feeling light

ignorance

having days off

Who Cares

sleep

camaraderie at work

your previous identity

the world making sense

sleep

walking side by side

not being someone people call strong

not needing to be strong

sleep

having less to explain

feeling in touch with the world

knowing what will come next

sleep

What you'll learn

the names of drugs

the opening hours of the hospital café

how to change a feeding tube

how to change an adult diaper

how to change

what to do when the incontinence service won't answer the phone

the glassy shine of a chemo scalp

the names of nurses

that god is deaf

who your friends are

Who Cares

how to moisten a mouth that can't drink

the parts of the body prone to sores

how to be invisible

how not to scream or cry

the weight of love

what happens one hundred miles past burnout

new forms of guilt

how to battle with bureaucracy

how to hide yourself deep, deep down

how to firefight

where in hospital there's phone signal, sometimes

where outside hospital there's a patch of sun, sometimes

the strange things people say as comfort

stoicism

desperation

the cocking of the head that says 'don't tell me too much'

how everyone thinks they'd do it better

how to break and still be standing

more patience than you ever thought you'd have

admiration for the others like you

What you'll need

sleep

sleep with your phone on silent

sleep with no risk of emergency

sleep without night terrors

sleep with a different world on waking

Who Cares

it all to end, but not to end

ibuprofen

money

bosses who understand

respite

other people who take true responsibility

training

therapy

to find the steel inside you

answered prayers

to believe you're planted, not buried

other people not to make you hold their discomfort for them

time

a time machine

your loved one not to be so sad

a map

a magic wand

to be able to breathe

someone to care for you, too

What you'll be

exhausted

angry

illuminated

Epilogue

In a conversation in the last months of her life, my mum mentioned a part of Wales called the Llŷn Peninsula and, more specifically, the wild island of Bardsey, two miles from the coast. I forget when she'd been there or why; bereavement is the slow drip of mundanities no longer knowable. But she told me I'd love it there, on that island. She knew I'd discovered a great passion for hiking by myself, for getting to know a country by the dogged placement of foot after foot. In July 2021, nearly a year after her death, I travelled to this place she'd told me I'd love. She was right. The peninsula was stunning in precisely the way I enjoy – rugged, wild and full of contrasts between bucolic vistas and jagged cliff edges. I loved every footstep. I saw blue butterflies for the first time, watched the bright red whizz of cinnabar moths amongst wildflowers, admired the jive of deep purple heather against sunny yellow gorse, and staved off heatstroke with impromptu dips in unpopulated coves, the water transparent and gloriously cool.

Mid-way through my hike around the coast, I took a ferry over to Bardsey Island, or Ynys Enlli as it's called by Welsh speakers, this place she'd especially recommended I seek out. The island has a rich history, and was a significant site for Celtic Christians who first built a monastery there in the sixth century. In the Middle Ages, it was said that three pilgrimages to Bardsey were equal to one to Rome. The ruins of a thirteenth-century abbey remain, grey, layered stones that tempt you to touch them, imagining those faithful forebears who trod the same ground. Bardsey also boasts puffins (much smaller in real life than you might expect) and seals that loll on the rocks, shiny and still as marble statues at first, then suddenly honking and flapping, making their blubber jiggle.

The island is tiny, less than a single square mile, and with a population of eleven people (and many sheep). I had thought being somewhere so small, where my footsteps would necessarily be on the same paths as hers had been, might provoke in me a rush of emotion. I had spent most of the previous year experiencing that 'formal feeling' that poet Emily Dickinson so astutely described as coming after great pain. And it did, indeed, feel strange to be standing somewhere so remote, and yet so small that I could be sure she'd stood in exactly this spot, marvelling at the same big blue out ahead or startled by the seals. I had intended that moment to be my allotted space for grief on my holiday. But grief has no interest in being project-managed. All I felt was a faint uncanniness, no rushing tears or gaping expiation.

The next day, I sat on the beach at nearby Llanbedrog, ensconced in the shade beneath the stone overhang of a bank behind me. A couple of elderly women and a man were to my right, a family with young kids to my left. I'd just eaten a clotted-cream ice cream (delicious). An elderly woman appeared in my line of vision, her direction of travel aimed at the group to my right. I couldn't look away from her. She was older than my mum, perhaps by a decade. And she looked very like how my mum might have looked, had she lived to that age, as if this woman on the beach was a ghost from an alternative future. She had the same body shape, before the distension of cancer and cachexia gave my mum that warped, saintly look of the dying. The ghost woman's hair was a brush on top of her head, like my mum's became after chemo turned it curly. And she walked with an unsteadiness that was never remotely how my mum walked – she of the high-heeled court shoes and smart suits, ready to rule the boardroom with a proud, imperious stride – but was also precisely the unsteadiness that came to characterise the sick woman who took my mum's place: less mother, more daughter, a confusing dissonance in a breaking body, once clever, but made naive by an unexpected journey for which she could grasp no map.

This woman, on the beach at Llanbedrog, the avatar of my mother's old age, walked with distracted pain across the burning sand to the people beside me. She held a folded metal deckchair in her left arm, its weight clearly on the brink of being too much. Such was the effort of the walk, the sand falling away in miniature sinking dunes at each step, that once she was a metre from us, her face took on the expression of slack confusion that comes with total exhaustion. I knew that look very well. Another thing I'd learned. I leapt up to relieve her of the chair, opening it and placing it down for her. She and her friends made cooing noises of gratitude. I nodded and looked back out to sea. I wondered

Who Cares

if they could tell from the twist of my mouth that the elderly woman was reminding me of someone. I sat back down and cried quietly for her, my mother; for the days by the sea she won't get, and that she would have loved.

Acknowledgements

I began writing the proposal for this book while my mother was still alive. She was terminally ill; I knew she would die, but I knew it thinly, like recalling the taste of something eaten a long time ago. Now I know it very differently. I hope she would be proud of this work, which has been both cathartic and wearying, and I hope she'd understand why I've told parts of our story. My first thank you is to her, for her quiet certitude in my writing abilities and dreams.

My thanks to my agent, Matthew Turner at RCW, for believing in my abilities and nurturing them, especially when my brain was half asleep amid bereavement. My thanks to Ella Gordon and Emma Berry, my wonderful wise duo of editors in the UK and USA respectively, and your excellent teams. I am beyond grateful to you all for your faith in me and in the significance of this topic. I believe many caregivers will be grateful to you, too.

To the Sisterhood, who once again find themselves in the pages of something I've written! Sophia, Carys, Jo, Fidi, Vicky, Jess, Lisa, Colette and Keelia, thank you for your kindnesses, for all our collective vulnerabilities and joys, and the nude rituals, too. For Amy Briggs, Susie Bennett, Sophie Hughes and Oli Harris, for cheerleading my writing endeavours over years past or present. Those moments of support exist simultaneously in the sheer audacity of sitting down to write each day.

For my mother's family members and friends, who knew sides of her I didn't and who miss her too. For my sister, whose acceptance of this project has been appreciated, and for the new path we're forging. For Nick and Lizzie, who provided blessed moments of respite from care and lost their sister, and especially for John, my mother's oldest brother, who died of cancer in January 2019. Before he was sick himself, he was a great help to us. My mum appreciated your presence so much, John: your long limbs tucked neatly into a hospital chair, reading a second-hand novel, while she fought, little knowing your own fight was on its way. I'm sorry for all of us in this family that there has been so much death and disease.

For every person who gave me their time for an interview: thank you, from me but also from every caregiver who reads your stories and finds solidarity. It wasn't just time you gave, but heartache and hope too. I hope I've done us all justice, and I am always out here, thinking of you. For the people who helped me access interviews, too – Anne Lise Sydnes, Martin Bakari, Maria Brenton and Sophie Otiende – thank you; it's these small actions that build bridges to better worlds.

Finally, for Richard. You are astonishing. Thank you for sitting with me by her side in the aftermath. Thank you for being half of our team in this ever-aftermath too. I love you.

Acknowledgements

I don't want to write the last words of these acknowledgements, because it marks an end to writing the story of me and her. This project has been a compass through the strange territories of grief, imposing sense on the senseless. Once again, I find myself at another closing of the door to her presence. I miss her. This is it.

Notes

Chapter 1 — On Caregivers: Missing Stories, Missing Solutions

1 Jane Jacobs. 1961. *The Death and Life of Great American Cities*, page 15.

2 Embracing Carers and the International Association of Carers Organization. 2021. *Global State of Caring*.

3 Eurocarers. 'About Carers'. eurocarers.org.

4 Family Caregiver Alliance. 'Caregiver Statistics: Demographics'. caregiver.org.

5 Jessica Moxham. 2021. *The Cracks that Let the Light In: What I Learned From My Disabled Son*. Endeavour, page 175.

6 Angela Stringfellow. 23 May 2017. 'Financial Support for Caregivers: The Ultimate Guide to Home Care Costs, Financial Aid, and Financial Planning for Caregivers'. Senior Link. seniorlink.com.

7 RAISE Family Caregiving Advisory Council. 2021. *Recognize, Assist, Include, Support, & Engage (RAISE) Family Caregivers Act: Initial Report to Congress*.

8 AARP Family Caregiving and National Alliance for Caregiving. 2020. *Caregiving in the US 2020*.

9 Evelyn Nakano Glenn. 2012. *Forced to Care: Coercion and Caregiving in America*. Harvard University Press, page 3.

10 Adrienne Rich. 2013. *The Dream of a Common Language*. W. W. Norton & Co., page 15.

11 Carers UK. 2017. *State of Caring Report 2017.*

12 Duane F. Stroman. 2003. *The Disability Rights Movement: From Deinstitutionalization to Self-Determination*. University Press of America, Inc. page 166.

13 Ibid, page 166.

14 Socialist Health Association. 1969. 'Chapter 13 of *Report on Ely Hospital*'. sochealth.co.uk.

15 Simon Jarrett. 2012. *Disability in Time and Place*. English Heritage Disability History, page 41.

16 Mark Smith. 23 March 2016. 'Untold stories from the notorious Ely Hospital are heard for the first time in a new exhibition'. Wales Online. walesonline.co.uk.

17 Jane Lewis. 1986. 'Introduction: Recognising Women's Experience of Home and Family'. In *Labour and Love: Women's Experience of Home and Family 1850–1940*. Ed. Jane Lewis. Basil Blackwell, page 3.

18 XinQi Dong, MD, MPH. 2016. 'Elder Rights in China: Care for Your Parents or Suffer Public Shaming and Desecrate Your Credit Scores'. *JAMA Internal Medicine*, Vol. 176, No. 10.

19 Vincent Ni. 31 May 2021. 'China announces three-child limit in major policy shift'. *Guardian*.

20 Takahiro Miyo. 2017. 'Why Do We Care for Old Parents? Evolutionary Genetic Model of Elderly Caring'. *Open Journal of Genetics*, Vol. 7, No. 1.

21 Jonathan Vespa. 13 March 2018. 'The Graying of American: More Older Adults Than Kids by 2035 – The U.S. Joins Other Countries With Large Aging Populations'. United States Census Bureau. census.gov.

22 University of Nottingham. 14 September 2018. 'New research suggests more than one in five children in England carry out some care for sick and disabled family members'. nottingham.ac.uk.

23 Carol Levine. 7 August 2017. 'More Than 1 Million Young Caregivers Live in the United States, But Policies Supporting Them Are Still "Emerging"'. Health Affairs. healthaffairs.org.

24 Melissa L. Caldwell. 2007. 'Elder Care in the New Russia: The Changing Face of Compassionate Social Security'. *European Journal of Anthropology*, Vol. 50, pages 72–3.

25 U.S. Department of Labor. 'Women in the Labor Force'. dol.gov; and Gill Court. 1995. *Women in the Labour Market: Two Decades of Change and Continuity*. Institute for Employment Studies.

26 Parkinson's Foundation. 10 July 2018. 'Parkinson's Foundation Prevalence Project Finds Number of People With Parkinson's Severely Underestimated'. parkinson.org.

27 Parkinson's UK. 2018. *The Incidence and Prevalence of Parkinson's in the UK: Results from the Clinical Practice Research Datalink Summary Report*. parkinsons.org.uk

28 Emiko Takagi, Adam Davey and Donna Wagner. 2013. 'A National Profile of Caregivers for the Oldest-Old'. *Journal of Comparative Family Studies*, Vol. 44.

29 Kimberly W. McDermott PhD, Anne Elixhauser PhD, and Ruirui Sun PhD. June 2017. 'Trends in Hospital Inpatient Stays in the United States, 2005–2014'. Agency for Healthcare Research and Equality. hcup-us.ahrq.gov; and OECD Data. 2021. 'Length of hospital stay'. data.oecd.org.

30 David Kendall. 2017. 'Creating a comprehensive strategy to support family caregivers'. Third Way. thirdway.org.

31 Emily Abel. 1991. *Who Cares for the Elderly?* Temple University Press, pages 91 and 99.

32 Evelyn Nakano Glenn. 2012. *Forced to Care: Coercion and Caregiving in America*. Harvard University Press, page 6.

33 Shu-Yuan Chao DNSc RN and Patricia Roth EdD RN. 2008. 'The experiences of Taiwanese women caring for parents-in-law'. *Journal of Advanced Nursing*, Vol.31, No. 3.

34 Socialstyrelsen. 2021. *Anhöriga som vårdar eller stödjer någon de står nära Underlag till en nationell strategi*. socialstyrelsen.se.

35 Embracing Carers. 2021. *Global Carer Wellbeing Index Report*.

36 Ibid.

37 Carers UK. 2020. *Unpaid carers twice as likely to have used a food bank during pandemic*. carersuk.org

Chapter 2 — On Women: Maidens and Migrants

1   Arvo Lindewall. 1925. 'Toveritar'. Reprinted in Varpu Lindström, "'I Won't Be a Slave!" – Finnish Domestics in Canada, 1911–30'. In Jean Burnet (ed.). 1986. *Looking into My Sister's Eyes: An Exploration in Women's History*. Multicultural History Society of Toronto.

2   Nakano Glenn. *Forced to Care*, pages 95–6.

3   Enobong Hannah Branch and Melissa E. Wooten. 2012. 'Suited for Service: Racialized Rationalizations for the Ideal Domestic Servant from the Nineteenth to the Early Twentieth Century'. *Social Science History*, Vol. 36, No. 2, page 170.

4   Ibid, page 171.

5   Jane Lewis. 1986. 'The Working-Class Wife and Mother and State Intervention, 1870–1918'. In *Labour and Love: Women's Experience of Home and Family 1850–1940*. Basil Blackwell.

6   Nakano Glenn. *Forced to Care*, page 97.

7   44Petra Ulmanen. 2017. *Family Care in the Swedish Welfare State: Extent, Content and Consequences*. Paper to the Transforming Care Conference. transforming-care.net.

8   OECD. 2021. 'Labour participation by sex and age'. oecd.org.

9   See also, Amani Karisa *et al.* 2021. '"Their status will be affected by that child": How masculinity influences father involvement in the education of learners with intellectual disabilities'. *Child: Care, Health and Development*, Vol. 47.

10 Nancy Folbre. 'The Care Penalty and Gender Inequality'. 2018. In *The Oxford Handbook of Women and the Economy*. Oxford University Press; and Sue Yeandle *et al.* 2007. 'Managing caring and employment'. University of Leeds and Carers UK.

11 Abel. *Who Cares for the Elderly?*, page 5.

12 Abel. *Who Cares for the Elderly?*, page 24.

13 Walter Simons. 2003. *Cities of Ladies: Beguine Communities in the Medieval Low Countries, 1200–1565*. University of Pennsylvania Press, page 74.

14 Christa Wichterich. 2020. 'Who Cares about Healthcare Workers? Care Extractivism and Care Struggles in Germany and India'. *Social Change*, Vol. 5, No. 1.

15 Businesswire. 23 February 2021. 'Global Adult Diaper Market Report 2021: A $24.2 Billion Market – Industry Trends, Share, Size, Growth, Opportunity and Forecast to 2026'. businesswire.com.

16 Richa Naidu. Undated. 'Adult incontinence market set to expand'. Reuters. fingfix.thomsonreuters.com

17 Coventry Patmore. 1858. *The Angel in the House.*

18 Dina. M. Copelman. 1986. 'A New Comradeship Between Men and Women: Family, Marriage and London's Women Teachers, 1870–1914.' In *Labour and Love: Women's experience of home and family 1850-1940*. Ed. Jane Lewis. Basil Blackwell, page 184.

19 See Jane Addams Digital Edition. Ramapo College. digital.janeaddams.ramapo.edu; and Abel. *Who Cares for the Elderly?*, page 39.

20 Nancy Fraser. 2016. 'Contradictions of Capital and Care'. *New Left Review.* newleftreview.org.

21 Angela Davis. 2019. *Women, Race and Class.* Penguin, page 209.

22 Carol Pateman. 2014. 'The Patriarchal Welfare State'. In Christopher Pierson *et al* (eds) *The Welfare State Reader*. Polity Press.

23 Ibid.

24 The Health Foundation. 20 March 1975. 'The Social Security Act 1975'. navigator.health.org.uk.

25 *Hansard*. 29 January 1975. 'Invalid Care Allowance'. House of Commons Deb. Vol. 885, cc562–9.

26 Pateman. 'The Patriarchal Welfare State', page 108.

27 Ibid.

28 Alix Kates Shulman and Honor Moore. 19 February 2021. 'A Brief History of Women's Liberation Movements in America'. Literary Hub. lithub.com.

29 Sisterhood and After Research Team. 8 March 2013. 'Women's Liberation: A National Movement'. British Library. bl.uk.

30 Nellie Bly. 1877. *Ten Days in a Mad-House.* University of Pennsylvania Digital Library. digital.library.upenn.edu.

31 Abel. *Who Cares for the Elderly?*, page 46.

32 Julia Wolfe et al. 14 May 2020. 'Domestic Workers Chartbook'. Economic Policiy Institute. epi.org.

33 O'Leary, Elizabeth L. 2003. *From Morning to Night*. University of Virginia Press.

34 Julie Kashen and Rakeen Mabud. July 2020. *Nevertheless, It Persists: Disrupting the Vicious Cycle of Institutionalized Sexism*. TIME'S UP Foundation. timesupfoundation.org.

35 Branch and Wooten. 'Suited for Service', page 179. 2012.

36 'The Gorilla Dissolution'. *The Big Bang Theory*. Directed by Peter Chakos. Season 7 Episode 23. Chuck Lorre Productions and Warner Bros.

37 Jeanne Batalova. 2018. 'Immigrant health-care workers in the United States'. Migration Policy Institute. migrationpolicy.org.

38 Dawn Lyon. 2006. 'The Organization of Care Work in Italy: Gender and Migrant Labor in the New Economy'. *Indiana Journal of Global Legal Studies*, Vol. 13, No. 1, page 218.

39 Amelita King-Dejardin. 2019. *The Social Construction of Migrant Care Work: At the Intersection of Care, Migration and Gender*. International Labour Organization. ilo.org.

40 Christa Wichterich. 2020. 'Who Cares about Healthcare Workers?'.

41 The term 'global care chains' was coined by: Arlie Hochschild. 2000. 'Global Care Chains and Emotional Surplus Value'. In *On the Edge: Living with Global Capitalism*. Jonathan Cape, pages 130–46.

42 TV Everyday. 2021. 'Me Before You – 27 February 2021 – Saturday – Channel 5'. tveveryday.com.

43 Nye Cominetti, Laura Gardiner and Gavin Kelly. 19 April 2020. 'What happens after the clapping finishes?' Resolution Foundation. resoutionfoundation.org; and Jennifer Gollan. 2020. 'Caregivers and takers'. Reveal. revealnews.org.

44 PHI. 2019. *U.S. Home Care Workers: Key Facts*. phinational.org.

45 Wichterich. 'Who Cares about Healthcare Workers?'

46 Virginia Eubanks and Alexandra Mateescu. 28 July 2021. '"We don't deserve this": new app places US caregivers under digital surveillance'. *Guardian*.

47 Ibid.

48 Yeandle *et al.* 'Managing Caring and Employment'.

49 Wichterich. 'Who Cares about Healthcare Workers?'

50 See Equal Care. equalcare.coop

51 See Emma Dowling. 2021. *The Care Crisis: What Caused It and How Can We End It?* Verso.

52 Morten Skovdal, Catherine Campbell and Vincent Onyango. 'Supporting "young carers" in Kenya: from policy paralysis to action'. *Childcare in Practice*, Vol. 19, No. 4.

53 Sophie Lewis. *Full Surrogacy Now: Feminism against Family.* Verso, page 76.

54 Joan Tronto. 1993. *Moral Boundaries: A Political Argument for an Ethic of Care.* Routledge.

55 Nancy Fraser. 1994. 'After the Family Wage: Gender Equity and the Welfare State'. *Political Theory*, Vol. 22, No. 4.

56 Nancy Fraser. 2013. *Fortunes of Feminism: From State-Managed Capitalism to Neoliberal Crisis.* Verso, page 33.

57 Ibid, page 133.

Chapter 3 — On Technology: Sleepwalking and Seal Pups

1 *Financial Times.* 2019. 'Robots/Ageing Japan: I, Carebot'. ft.com.

2 Eugene Demaitre. 17 January 2019. 'ElliQ Social Companion Robot Aimed at Elders Now Available for Preorder'. Robotics Business Review. roboticsbusinessreview.com.

3 Ibid.

4 ElliQ. elliq.com.

5 Ibid.

6 Moxham. *The Cracks that Let the Light In*, page 22.

7 'About'. Ageless Innovation. agelessinnovation.com

8 'Companion Pet Cats'. Joy for All. joyforall.com

9 Malcolm Foster. 28 March 2018. 'Aging Japan: Robots may have role in future of elder care'. Reuters. reuters.com.

10   WIRED. 30 March 2015. 'Huggable robot befriends girl in hospital' [video]. youtube.com.

11   Shoshanna Solomon. 13 February 2020. 'Israeli social companion robot ElliQ gets added funding boost'. *Times of Israel.*

12   'Robots/Ageing Japan'.

13   Foster. 'Aging Japan'.

14   National Science Foundation. 8 September 2021. 'NRI/Collaborative Research: Robot-Assisted Feeding: Towards Efficient, Safe, and Personalized Caregiving Robots'. nsf.gov; and National Science Foundation. 15 September 2018. 'NRI: FND: Controllable Compliance: A New Robotic Arm for Contact-Rich Manipulation'. nsf.gov; and National Science Foundation. 11 August 2020. 'NRI: FND: Assistive Child-Robot Interventions for Infants with Motor Disabilities'. nsf.gov.

15   Department for Business, Energy and Industrial Strategy. 26 October 2019. 'Care robots could revolutionise UK care system and provide staff extra support'. gov.uk.

16   Shadow Robots. 17 April 2018. 'Our sincere thanks to our partners'. www.shadowrobot.com.

17   University of the West of England. 4 December 2015. 'Innovate UK funding for assistive robotic system will offer a "new perspective on ageing"'info.uwe.ac.uk.

18   Aimee van Wynsberghe. 2013. 'Designing Robots for Care: Care Centered Value-Sensitive Design'. *Science and Engineering Ethics*, Vol. 19.

19   Gary Chan Kok Yew. 2021. Trust in and Ethical Design of Carebots: The Case for Ethics of Care. *International Journal of Social Robotics*, Vol. 13.

20   Winner. L. (1983) Technologies as forms of life. In Epistemology, Methodology and the Social Sciences, eds. Cohen and Wartofsky. Kluwer Academic Publishers.

21   'About Us'. Just Checking. justchecking.co.uk.

22   AKTIVE Consortium. 2013. *The Role of Telecare in Meeting the Needs of Older People.* The Oxford Institute of Population Ageing. ageing.ox.ac.uk.

23 Ibid.

24 Aspect, 2020. *Caring During Lockdown: Challenges and Opportunities for Digitally Supporting Carers.* Centre for International Research on Care, Labour and Equalities. circle. group.shef.ac.uk.

25 'PARO Therapeutic Robot'. parorobots.com.

26 Lillian Hung *et al.* 2019. 'The benefits of and barriers to using a social robot PARO in care settings: a scoping review'. *BMC Geriatrics*, Vol. 19.

27 Ibid.

28 Ibid.

29 Ibid.

30 BBC News. 28 December 2021. 'Alexa tells 10-year-old girl to touch live plug with penny'. bbc.co.uk/news; and Kristin Livdahl [@ klivdahl]. 26 December 2021. 'OMFG My 10 year old just asked Alexa on our Echo for a challenge and this is what she said' [Tweet]. twitter.com.

31 National Robotics Initiative. 31 October 2016. *A Roadmap for US Robotics: From Internet to Robotics, 2016 Edition.* Computing Research Association. cra.org.

32 Kory Floyd. 31 August 2013. 'What lack of affection can do to you'. *Psychology Today.* psychologytoday.com.

33 Kory Floyd. 2016. 'Affection deprivation is associated with physical pain and poor sleep quality'. *Communication Studies*, Vol. 67, No. 4.

34 Colin Hesse *et al.* 2021. 'Affection deprivation during the COVID-19 pandemic: A panel study'. *Journal of Social and Personal Relationships*, Vol. 38, No. 10; and Floyd. 'Affection deprivation is associated with physical pain and poor sleep quality'.

35 Korisky *et al.* 2020. 'A dual-brain approach for understanding the neural mechanisms that underlie the comforting effects of social touch'. *Cortex*, Vol. 127.

36 Shannon Vallor. 2011. 'Carebots and Caregivers: Sustaining the Ethical Ideal of Care in the Twenty-First Century'. *Philosophy and Technology*, Vol. 24.

37 Wynsberghe. 'Designing Robots for Care'.

Chapter 4 — On Family: Wise Women and the Practice of Kinning

1   Bue Rübner Hansen and Manuela Zechner. 2019. 'Extending the family: reflections on the politics of kinship'. In Camille Barbagallo *et al* (eds). *Commoning with George Caffentzis and Silvia Federici*. Pluto Press.

2   AARP and NAC. *Caregiving in the US 2020*; and Carers UK. 2021. *State of Caring Report 2021*.

3   Tomas Frejka. 11 December 2017. 'Half the world's population is reaching below replacement fertility'. Institute for Family Studies. ifstudies.org.

4   Laura Wamsley. 24 December 2019. 'Japan's births decline to lowest on record'. NPR. npr.org.

5   Clare Ansberry. 20 July 2018. 'America Is Running Out of Family Caregivers, Just When It Needs Them Most'. *Wall Street Journal.* wsj.com.

6   James Lloyd. October 2008. *The State of Intergenerational Relations Today.* International Longevity Centre. ilcuk.org.

7   Natalie Campisi. 14 December 2020. '"Grannie units" are all the rage as multigenerational households grow'. Realty One Group. realtyonegroup.com.

8   Walter Simons. 2001. *Cities of Ladies: Beguine Communities in the Medieval Low Countries 1200–1565*. University of Pennsylvania Press, page 7.

9   Institutions for Collective Action. 'The European Marriage Pattern'. collective-action.info.

10 Tine de Moor. 2014. 'Single, Safe, and Sorry?: Explaining the Early Modern Beguine Movement in the Low Countries'. *Journal of Family History*, Vol. 39, No. 1.

11 Anna Muraco. 2006. 'Intentional Families: Fictive Kin Ties between Cross-Gender, Different Sexual Orientation Friends'. *Journal of Marriage and Family*, Vol. 68, No. 5.

12 Michele Barrett and Mary Mcintosh. 1982. The Antisocial Family.

13 Andrew Nocon and Maggie Pearson. 2000. 'The roles of friends

and neighbours in providing support for older people'. *Ageing and Society*, Vol. 20.

14 Isabelle Rey-Lefebvre. 16 Feburary 2016. 'Mort de la militante féministe Thérèse Clerc'. *Le Monde*. lemonade.fr.

15 Cat Johnson. 2016. 'Aging in the community: Inside the senior cohousing community'. Shareable. shareable.net.

16 New Ground Cohousing. owch.org.uk.

17 Spruil *et al.* 2014. 'Non-Biological (Fictive Kin and Othermothers): Embracing the Need for a Culturally Appropriate Pedigree Nomenclature in African-American Families'. *Journal of the National Black Nurses Association*, Vol. 25, No. 2.

18 Ibid.

19 Elizabeth Brake. 2013. 'Recognizing care: the case for friendship and polyamory'. *Syracuse Journal of Law and Civic Engagement*, Issue 1.

Chapter 5 — On the Mind: Confronting a Convenient Stigma

1 George Bataille.1986. *Eroticism: Death and Sensuality*. City Lights Books, page 15.

2 Carers UK forum post.

3 Ibid.

4 Ibid.

5 Beth Perry *et al.* 2010. 'Family caregivers' compassion fatigue in long-term facilities: a Canadian study offers staff in the UK insight into the feelings of hopelessness and sadness that can engulf relatives assisting with care, say Beth Perry and colleagues'. *Nursing Older People*, Vol. 22, No. 4.

6 Carers UK forum post.

7 Mary Mullenbach and Thomas M. Skovholt. 2016. 'Burnout prevention and self-care strategies of expert practitioners'. In *The Resilient Practitioner: Burnout and compassion fatigue prevention and self-care strategies for the helping professions*. Routledge.

8   Carers UK forum post.

9   Caring.com. '80% of Caregivers Report Strain on Their Marriages'. 2009. caring.com.

10   Linda Fodrini-Johnson. 2010. 'My marriage or my mom!' *Aging Well*, Vol. 3, No. 3; and Annalisa Barbieri. 2021. 'Is my marriage over or am I just exhausted from caring for my mum?' *Guardian*.

11   Caring.com. '80% of Caregivers Report Strain on Their Marriages'.

12   David R. Hodge and Fei Sun. 2012. 'Positive feelings of caregiving among Latino Alzheimer's family caregivers: Understanding the role of spirituality'. *Aging and Mental Health*, Vol. 16, No. 6.

13   Mark Schaller *et al.* 2003. 'Prehistoric dangers and contemporary prejudices'. *European Review of Social Psychology*, Vol. 14, No. 1; and Oaten *et al.* 2011. 'Disease avoidance as a functional basis for stigmatization'. *Philosophical Transactions of the Royal Society of London B: Biological Sciences*, Vol. 366, No. 1583.

14   Schaller *et al.* 'Prehistoric dangers and contemporary prejudices'.

15   Oaten *et al.* 2011. 'Disease avoidance as a functional basis for stigmatization'.

16   Ibid.

17   Imogen Tyler. 2020. *Stigma: The Machinery of Inequality.* Zed Books.

18   Papadopoulos *et al.* 2018. 'Systematic review of the relationship between autism stigma and informal caregiver mental health'. *Journal of Autism and Developmental Disorders*, Vol. 49, No. 4.

19   Korschorke *et al.* 2017. 'Experiences of stigma and discrimination faced by family caregivers of people with schizophrenia in India'. *Social Science and Medicine*, Vol. 178.

20   Erving Goffman. 1963. *Stigma: Notes on the Management of Spoiled Identity.* Penguin, page 47.

21   Cambridge Dictionary online. 'Evolution'. dictionary.cambridge. org.

22   Cited in Sheldon Solomon, Jeff Greenberg and Tom Pyszczynski. 2015. *The Worm at the Core: On the Role of Death in Life.* Allen Lane, page 218.

Chapter 6 — On Freedom: The Lie of the Individual

1   Lisa Robinson. September 2010. 'Lady Gaga's Cultural Revolution'. *Vanity Fair.*

2   Simone de Beauvoir. 1949. *The Second Sex.* Vintage Books, page 98.

3   Tronto. *Moral Boundaries*, page 163.

4   United Nations Economic and Social Commission for Asia and the Pacific. 2019. *Unpaid Work in Asia and the Pacific.* UN ESCAP, page 23.

5   Hope Landrine. 1992. 'Clinical implications of cultural differences: The referential versus the indexical self'. *Clinical Psychology Review.* Vol. 12, No. 4, page 404.

6   Ibid, page 403.

7   Martha Nussbaum. 2000. 'The Future of Feminist Liberalism'. *Proceedings and Addresses of the American Philosophical Association*, Vol. 74, No. 2.

8   Cynthia Griffith. 14 June 2021. '59% of Americans are just one paycheck away from homelessness'. Invisible People. invisiblepeople.tv.

9   Alasdair Sandford. 3 April 2020. 'Coronavirus: Half of humanity now on lockdown as 90 countries call for confinement'. Euronews. euronews.com.

10   Zoe Wood and Sarah Butler. 12 March 2020. 'Coronavirus triggers sharp rise in price of pain relief medication'. *Guardian.*

11   Julia Robinson. 2020. 'Paracetamol sold for more than £50 per tablet on online bidding sites'. *The Pharmaceutical Journal.* pharmaceutical-journal.com.

12   Leanne Italie and Jessie Wardarski. 18 March 2020. 'Two 20-somethings extend "invisible hands" in virus outbreak'. AP News. apnews.com; and Tsai City. 13 May 2020. 'Invisible Hands Deliver: Talking innovation and grassroots impact with Liam Elkind'. medium.com; and Lisa Kava. 10 January 2022. 'Invisible Hands expands to deliver free groceries'. West Side Rag. westsiderag.com.

13   'Village Model'. Village to Village Network. vtvnetwork.org.

14 Rebecca Solnit. 14 May 2020. "'The way we get through this is together": the rise of mutual aid under coronavirus'. *Guardian.*

15 Phillip Hollobone. *Hansard.* 22 July 2021. 'Support for carers'. House of Commons Deb. Vol. 699.

16 Margaret Walker, quoted in Virginia Held. 2005. *The Ethics of Care: Personal, Political and Global.* Oxford University Press.

17 María Puig de la Bellacasa. 2017. *Matters of Care: Speculative Ethics in More Than Human Worlds.* Minnesota University Press. Kindle edition.

Chapter 7 — On Work: Breadwinners and Caregivers

1   Philip Larkin. 1955. 'Toads'. In *The Less Deceived.* Faber and Faber.

2   Family Caregiving Alliance. 'Caregiver Statistics: Work and Caregiving'. caregiver.org.

3   CIPD. June 2020. *Supporting Working Carers: How Employers and Employees Can Benefit.* 2020. http://www.cipd.co.uk/Images/supporting-working-carers-2_tcm18-80339.pdf CIPD and the University of Sheffield. cipd.co.uk.

4   Tronto. *Moral Boundaries*, page 165.

5   Working Families. 2018. *2018 Off Balance: Parents of Disabled Children and Paid Work.* workingfamilies.org.uk.

6   Fraser. 'Contradictions of Capital and Care'.

7   Michael Hoffman. 12 September 2010. 'Ageing through the ages'. *Japan Times.* japantimes.co.jp.

8   Tim G. Parkin. 2004. *Old Age in the Roman World: A Cultural and Social History.* JHUP.

9   Apolitical. 22 October 2018. 'How will technology change care work?' apolitical.co.

10 Amazon Staff. 21 August 2020. 'Amazon offers back-up care to 650,000 US employees'. Amazon. aboutamazon.com.

11 BBC News. 6 July 2021. 'Four-day week "an overwhelming success" in Iceland'. bbc.co.uk/news.

12 Laurie Havelock. 26 January 2022. 'A four-day working week sounds like a dream come true, but it could soon be how we all work'. iNews. inews.co.uk.

13 BBC Bitesize. 'Who invented the weekend?'. bbc.co.uk/bitesize.

14 Li-Mei Chen and Konomi Imai. 2013. 'Female Informal Caregivers in Sweden and Implications for Japan: A Feminist Perspective'. *Social Sciences Review*, Vol. 18.

15 Margunn Bjørnholt. 2014. 'Changing men, changing times – fathers and sons from an experimental gender equality study'. *The Sociological Review*, Vol. 62.

16 Peter Cynkar and Elizabeth Mendes. 26 July 2011. 'More than one in six American workers also act as caregivers'. Gallup-Healthways. news.gallup.com.

17 Family Caregiving Alliance. 'Caregiver Statistics: Work and Caregiving'.

18 Scott Brown *et al.* 2020. *Employee and Worksite Perspectives of the Family and Medical Leave Act: Executive Summary for Results from the 2018 Surveys.* Abt Associates and the Department of Labor. dol.gov.

19 Ibid.

20 The White House. 21 September 2021. 'FACT SHEET: How the Build Back Better Framework Will Support the Sandwich Generation'. whitehouse.gov.

21 Paying for Senior Care. 5 November 2020. 'New York paid family leave benefits law and caring for the elderly'. payingforseniorcare.com.

22 The White House. 'FACT SHEET: How the Build Back Better Framework Will Support the Sandwich Generation'; and Kelly-Anne Smith and Lisa Rowan. 20 December 2021. 'Manchin Drops Support For Build Back Better. What's Next For Biden's Big Social Plan?'. Forbes. forbes.com.

23 UK Government. 'Time off for family and dependants'. gov.uk.

24 'The Netherlands: Eurocarers Country Profiles'. eurocarers.org.

25 'Eurocarers Country Profiles'. eurocarers.org

26 European Commission: Employment, Social Affairs and Inclusion. 'Work-Life Balance'. ec.europa.eu; and European Commission.

26 April 2017. 'Document 52017DC0252 – Communication from the Commission to the European Parliament, the Council, the European Economic and Social Committee and the Committee of the Regions: An Initiative to Support Work-Life Balance for Working Parents and Carers'. EUR-Lex. eur-lex.europa.eu.

27　Alexandra Toppin. 26 April 2021. 'Shared parental leave: scrap 'deeply flawed' policy say campaigners'. *Guardian*.

28　Sweden. 'Equal power and influence for women and men'. sweden.se.

29　CIPD. 2019. *Megatrends: Flexible Working*. cipd.co.uk.

30　Janet Hook and Peter Wallsten. 6 August 2004. 'President pushes flextime'. *Los Angeles Times*. latimes.com.

31　OECD. September 2016. *Be Flexible! Background Brief on How Workplace Flexibility Can Help European Employees to Balance Work and Family*. oecd.org.

32　Cynthia Thomas Calvert. 2016. *Caregivers in the Workplace: Family Responsibilities Litigation Update 2016*. WorkLifeLaw. worklifelaw.org.

33　Taylor Hatmaker. 8 February 2017. 'Facebook announces paid family sick leave and new bereavement benefits for employees'. Tech Crunch. techcrunch.com.

34　*Northwestern and Care@Work: Working Together to Make Adult Care a Strategic Employee Benefit*. Northwestern University and Care@Work.

35　Portable Benefits. 10 November 2015. 'Common ground for independent workers'. WTF Economy. wtfeconomy.com.

36　Joseph B. Fuller and Manjari Raman. 2019. *The Caring Company: How Employers Can Help Their Employees Manage Their Caregiving Responsibilities – While Reducing Costs and Increasing Productvity*. Harvard Business School.

37　See Carer Passport. carerpassport.uk.

38　Mandy Cook. November 2020. *Policy and Practice Brief: Support for employees who combine paid work with unpaid care: 2*. Centre for International Research on Care, Labour and Equalities (CIRCLE). circle.group.shef.ac.uk.

39　Bronnie Ware. 2012. The Top Five Regrets of the Dying: A Life Transformed by the Dearly Departing. Hay House UK.

Chapter 8 — On Government: Commoning the Horizon

1 J. K. Gibson-Graham. *A Postcapitalist Politics*. 2006. Minnesota University Press, page 127.
2 The White House. 28 October 2021. 'Remarks by President Biden Announcing the Framework for His Build Back Better Agenda and Bipartisan Infrastructure Bill'. whitehouse.gov.
3 Kirsten Gillibrand [@SenGillibrand]. 7 April 2021. 'Paid leave is infrastructure. Child care is infrastructure. Caregiving is infrastructure' [Tweet]. twitter.com.
4 Ibid: replies.
5 Ibid: replies.
6 Danielle Kurtzleben. 15 April 2021. 'What is infrastructure?' NPR. npr.org.
7 The White House. 28 October 2021. 'Remarks by President Biden Announcing the Framework for His Build Back Better Agenda and Bipartisan Infrastructure Bill'. whitehouse.gov.
8 Tony Abraham. 14 September 2018. 'When ICE comes knocking, healthcare workers want to be prepared.' Healthcare Dive. healthcaredive.com.
9 Hatem Mona *et al.* 2021. 'Barriers to accessing health care among undocumented migrants in Sweden – a principal component analysis'. *BMC Health Services Research*, Vol. 21.
10 Community Catalysts. 17 July 2019. 'It's time for local area coordination'. communitycatalysts.co.uk.
11 Patrick Butler. 27 August 2015. 'Thousands died after fit for work assessment'. *Guardian;* and Laura Pidcock. 24 April 2019. *Hansard.* 'Ten Years of the Work Capability Assessment'. House of Commons Deb. Vol. 658.
12 Inclusive Neighbourhoods. 'What is local area coordination?'. inclusiveneighbourgoods.co.uk.
13 RAISE Family Caregiving Advisory Council. *(RAISE) Family Caregivers Act.*
14 Ibid.

15 Joseph Guzman. 9 October 2020. 'Researchers surprised by experiment that gave homeless people thousands of dollars'. The Hill. thehill.com.

16 David Bollier and Silke Helfrich. 2019. *Free, Fair and Alive: The Insurgent Power of the Commons.* New Society Publishers.

17 David Bollier. 2016. 'A Report on a Deep Dive Workshop convened by the Commons Strategies Group in cooperation with the Heinrich Böll Foundation'. Commons Strategies Group. commonsstrategies.org.

18 Silvia Federici. 2012. *Revolution at Point Zero: Housework, Reproduction and Feminist Struggle.* PM Press, page 21.

19 Silke Helfrich. 8 September 2021. 'WSI Announcements 5/2021'. commons.blog.

20 Federici. *Revolution at Point Zero,* page 125.

Conclusion

1 Mary Gaitskill. 2021. *Oppositions: Selected Essays.* Serpent's Tail..

2 'Alcor – Extend your life with cyronics'. alcor.org; and Zack Guzman. 26 April 2016. 'This company will freeze your dead body for $200,000'. NBC News. nbcnews.com.

3 Charles Darwin. 1871. *The Descent of Man,* page 492.

4 Sheldon Solmon *et al.* 2015. *The Worm at the Core: On the Role of Death in Life.* Penguin, page viii.

5 Ibid, page 39.

6 Ibid, page 225.

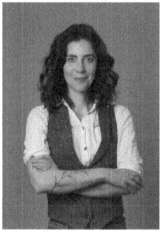

© Susan Torkington

Emily Kenway is a writer, activist and former policy advisor. Her first book, *The Truth About Modern Slavery*, was published in 2021. She has written for a variety of publications including the *Guardian, Independent, OpenDemocracy, Huffington Post, Litro* and *TLS*. Her non-fiction has been nominated for a Pushcart Prize, and in 2020 she was shortlisted for the Alpine Fellowship Writing Prize. *Who Cares*, her second book, will publish in spring 2023.